CLINICAL CHALLENGES IN HYPERTENSION II

CLINICAL CHALLENGES IN HYPERTENSION II

Edited by

Peter P. Toth
Director of Preventive Cardiology, Sterling Rock Falls Clinic
Chief of Medicine, CGH Medical Center, Sterling, Illinois
Clinical Associate Professor, University of Illinois College of Medicine,
Peoria, Illinois, Southern Illinois University School of Medicine
Springfield, Illinois, USA

Domenic Sica
Professor of Medicine and Pharmacology
Chairman, Clinical Pharmacology and Hypertension, Division of
Nephrology, Virginia Commonwealth University Health System
Richmond, Virginia, USA

CLINICAL PUBLISHING

OXFORD

Clinical Publishing
an imprint of Atlas Medical Publishing Ltd

Oxford Centre for Innovation
Mill Street, Oxford OX2 0JX, UK
Tel: +44 1865 811116
Fax: +44 1865 251550
Email: info@clinicalpublishing.co.uk
Web: www.clinicalpublishing.co.uk

Distributed in USA and Canada by:
Clinical Publishing
30 Amberwood Parkway
Ashland OH 44805, USA
Tel: 800-247-6553 (toll free within US and Canada)
Fax: 419-281-6883
Email: order@bookmasters.com

Distributed in UK and Rest of World by:
Marston Book Services Ltd
PO Box 269
Abingdon
Oxon OX14 4YN, UK
Tel: +44 1235 465500
Fax: +44 1235 465555
Email: trade.orders@marston.co.uk

A catalogue record for this book is available from the British Library

ISBN 13   978 1 84692 069 1
ISBN e-book   978 1 84692 621 1

Project manager: Gavin Smith, GPS Publishing Solutions, Hertfordshire, UK
Typeset by Mizpah Publishing Services Private Limited, Chennai, India
Printed by Marston Book Services Ltd, Abingdon, Oxon, UK

Contents

Editors

PETER P. TOTH, MD, PhD, FAAFP, FICA, FNLA, FCCP, FAHA, FACC, Director of Preventive Cardiology, Sterling Rock Falls Clinic; Chief of Medicine, CGH Medical Center, Sterling, Illinois; Clinical Associate Professor, University of Illinois College of Medicine, Peoria, Illinois, Southern Illinois University School of Medicine, Springfield, Illinois, USA

DOMENIC SICA, MD, Professor of Medicine and Pharmacology; Chairman, Clinical Pharmacology and Hypertension, Division of Nephrology, Virginia Commonwealth University Health System, Richmond, Virginia, USA

Contributors

GEORGE L. BAKRIS, MD, HonD, FASN, FAHA, Professor of Medicine, Director, Hypertensive Diseases Unit, University of Chicago, Pritzker School of Medicine, Chicago, Illinois, USA

JAN BASILE, MD, Professor of Medicine, Seinsheimer Cardiovascular Health Program, Division of General Internal Medicine/Geriatrics, Medical University of South Carolina, Research Associate, Primary Care Service Line, Ralph H. Johnson VA Medical Center, Charleston, South

BASIL BURNEY, MD, Fellow in Hypertension, University of Chicago, Pritzker School of Medicine, Chicago, Illinois, USA

BARRY L. CARTER, PharmD, FCCP, FAHA, Professor, Department of Pharmacy Practice and Science, College of Pharmacy and Department of Family Medicine, College of Medicine, University of Iowa, Iowa City, Iowa, USA

STEVEN L. DUBOVSKY, MD, Professor and Chair, Department of Psychiatry, University at Buffalo, Departments of Psychiatry and Medicine, University of Colorado, Buffalo, New York, USA

MICHAEL E. ERNST, PharmD, FCCP, Professor (Clinical), Department of Pharmacy Practice and Science, College of Pharmacy and Department of Family Medicine, College of Medicine, University of Iowa, Iowa City, Iowa, USA

JOHN M. FLACK, MD, MPH, FAHA, FACP, FACSG, Chairman, Department of Medicine; Chief, Division of Translational Research and Clinical Epidemiology, Wayne State University, Detroit Medical Center, Detroit, Michigan, USA

DONNA S. HANES, MD, Associate Professor of Medicine, Division of Nephrology, University of Maryland Hospital, Baltimore, Maryland, USA

JOSEPH L. IZZO JR., MD, FACP, FAHA, Professor of Medicine, Professor of Pharmacology and Toxicology, Clinical Director of Medicine, State University of New York at Buffalo, School of Medicine and Biomedical Sciences and the Erie County Medical Center, Buffalo, NY, USA

NITHIN KARAKALA, MD, Internal Medicine Resident, St Agnes Hospital, Baltimore, Maryland, USA

JANE MORLEY KOTCHEN, MD, MPH, Professor, Departments of Population Health and Medicine, Medical College of Wisconsin, Milwaukee, Wisconsin, USA

THEODORE A. KOTCHEN, MD, MBA, Professor of Medicine, Medical College of Wisconsin, Milwaukee, Wisconsin, USA

JOHN J. LEDDY, MD, FACSM, FACP, Associate Professor of Clinical Orthopaedics, Assistant Professor of Medicine, Family Medicine, Rehabilitation Sciences and Nutrition, Research Assistant Professor of Physiology, University Sports Medicine, State University of New York at Buffalo, School

WILLIAM B. MOSKOWITZ, MD, FAAP, FACC, FSCAI, Professor, Pediatrics and Internal Medicine; Chair, Pediatric Cardiology; Director, Pediatric Cardiac Catheterization Laboratory; Vice Chair, Department of Pediatrics, Children's Medical Center, Medical College of Virginia, Virginia Commonwealth Universit

JAMES L. POOL, MD, Professor of Medicine and Pharmacology, Baylor College of Medicine, Houston, Texas, USA

SHAKAIB U. REHMAN, MD, FACP, FAACH, Chief of Primary Care, Associate Professor of Medicine, Ralph H. Johnson VA Medical Center, Medical University of South Carolina, Charleston, South Carolina, USA

ADDISON A. TAYLOR, MD, PhD, Professor of Medicine and Pharmacology, Division of Hypertension and Clinical Pharmacology, Section on Cardiovascular Research, Department of Medicine, Baylor College of Medicine, Houston, Texas, USA

DONALD G. VIDT, MD, Emeritus Chairman/Consultant, Department of Hypertension and Nephrology, Cleveland Clinic, Cleveland, Ohio, USA

CALVERT WARREN, MD, Assistant Professor and Director of Psychiatric Emergency Services, Department of Psychiatry, University at Buffalo, Departments of Psychiatry and Medicine, University of Colorado, Buffalo, New York, USA

MATTHEW R. WEIR, MD, Professor and Director, Division of Nephrology, University of Maryland School of Medicine, Baltimore, Maryland, USA

Foreword

Hypertension is the most common form of cardiovascular disease in economically developed and developing countries, afflicting over 73 million persons in the US and over one billion worldwide. Left uncontrolled, it is a major contributor to death and disability due to stroke, coronary artery disease and chronic kidney disease. While blood pressure reduction has been shown in randomized controlled trials to be highly effective in preventing acute cardiovascular events and death, attainment of guideline specified blood pressure goals in the practice setting has proved difficult. Much of the difficulty experienced by primary care providers and hypertension specialists alike in managing blood pressure comes from conflicting information about the relative efficacy of various antihypertensive measures, both pharmacologic and nonpharmacologic (lifestyle modification). Further, there is a paucity of authoritative information about how to approach blood pressure management in patients with comorbidities that may be driving blood pressure elevation (anxiety and panic disorders, sleep disorders, athletic activities) or that may limit therapeutic choices (acute and chronic stroke, coronary artery disease) and in special patient populations (adolescents and young adults, the very elderly).

Edited by preventive cardiologist Peter Toth and clinical pharmacologist Domenic Sica, this new book fulfils an urgent need of those who care for hypertensive patients by providing answers or at least approaches to practical questions that are not addressed in current guidelines. The volume is organized around frequently asked questions about hypertension that surface time and time again at educational symposia. Issues discussed include both core clinical and scientific concepts and practical everyday patient related issues that are not well covered in most hypertension guidelines.

Chapters by world experts offer advice on such critical questions as: How should we use home (self) blood pressure measurement vs. 24 hour ambulatory blood pressure monitoring vs. office-based blood pressure readings for diagnosis and management of hypertension? What are appropriate treatment goals for systolic and diastolic blood pressure? In what patient groups? Does lifestyle modification play a major-and sustainable-role in hypertension management? If pharmacologic therapy is needed, does it matter what we use? Should we believe, as stated in JNC7, that diuretic therapy should be first step therapy in all (or nearly all) hypertensive patients? Or, should we adopt the recommendations of the more recent European guidelines that several classes of antihypertensive drugs are appropriate for first line treatment, at the discretion of the caregiver? What is more important, getting to goal blood pressure or blocking critical pathways, e.g., the renin-angiotensin-aldosterone system? In other words, when considering antihypertensive treatment, does mechanism matter? Are all angiotensin converting enzyme (ACE) inhibitors equally effective in lowering blood pressure? Protecting target organs? Are angiotensin receptor blockers (ARBs) equivalent or superior to ACE inhibitors in controlling blood pressure and protecting target organs? What is the best way to treat morning surges in blood pressure?

Importantly, there are many hypertensive patients for whom treatment recommendations based on the strongest form of evidence, the randomized controlled trial, are lacking. Chapters in this book address many of these common and difficult to manage situations, e.g. the patient with anxiety/panic disorder and labile hypertension, the post-stroke (both acute and chronic) patient, the athlete who wishes to continue to compete despite his/her hypertension, the adolescent or young adult with hypertension in whom the short term risk of cardiovascular disease/events is low but the long term prognosis may not be benign, and the patient with a hypertensive emergency. For many of these conditions, there may never be randomized controlled trial data. In the meantime, the caregiver must rely on expert opinion and his/her own experience in caring for patients with these complex problems. *Clinical Challenges in Hypertension II* (along with its companion volume *Challenges in Hypertension*) is a treasure trove of valuable expert opinion on how to deal with many important problems in hypertension management. I recommend it highly.

Suzanne Oparil, MD
Professor of Medicine, Physiology & Biophysics
Director, Vascular Biology and Hypertension Program
Cardiovascular Disease
Department of Medicine
University of Alabama at Birmingham

Preface

Hypertension (HTN) is a complex, multifactorial disease. In the last four decades an enormous amount of experimental, epidemiologic, and clinical investigation has demonstrated beyond all doubt that elevations in both systolic and diastolic blood pressure exert deleterious effects on the vasculature. Progressive injury stemming from chronically elevated blood pressure increases risk for developing endothelial dysfunction, loss of vascular elasticity and distensibility, atherosclerosis, left ventricular hypertrophy, heart failure, ischemic and hemorrhagic stroke, peripheral arterial disease, as well as proteinuria and nephropathy. Hypertension is widely prevalent throughout the world and constitutes a significant public health issue. The incidence of HTN is increasing in men and women and in people across all ethnic groups.

The treatment of hypertension is one of the true cornerstones in any approach to reducing risk for cardiovascular events in both the primary and secondary prevention settings. Evidence-based, population specific guidelines for the treatment of HTN have been developed by numerous expert bodies. These guidelines are rigorous and based on many well done prospective, randomized clinical trials. They emphasize the critical need to lower elevated blood pressure with lifestyle modification and pharmacologic intervention and to treat patients with end organ injury with specific classes of drugs. Despite the clarity and utility of many of these guidelines, there continues to be low rates of attaining target blood pressure in approximately two-thirds of the patients with HTN. Clearly, more focused efforts at improving the identification and management of HTN need to be implemented. Patient compliance and access to medication must also be improved.

The etiology of HTN depends on specific, highly complex genetic and metabolic backgrounds. Environmental influences (e.g. social/psychological stress, salt intake, diet) also play significant roles. The brain, kidney, and visceral adipose tissue regulate a wide range of biochemical and physiological responses which intimately influence the molecular and histologic dynamics of arterial walls, leading to increased vasomotor tone and HTN.

Hypertension in any given individual is often multifactorial. During the last 60 years, many different drug classes have been developed to antagonize specific mechanisms by which blood pressure is raised (i.e. reducing intravascular volume, inhibiting renin and angiotensin converting enzyme, blocking intravascular catecholamine and angiotensin II receptors, and blocking calcium channels in smooth muscle cells). The majority of patients require combinations of drugs to control their blood pressure, especially in the presence of end organ damage. It requires clinical experience and insight into drug mechanisms to appropriately target specific mechanisms with specific drugs in order to optimally control blood pressure.

There are numerous fine textbooks in the field of hypertension and nephrology. This book is not intended to be encyclopedic. Rather, it is framed as a series of questions with detailed answers that are as evidence-based as possible. The authors are all experts in the field of HTN management. The questions posed are those that often arise at major conferences. These are the sorts of questions that often puzzle clinicians the most, or leave them wondering what the evidence supporting certain approaches really consists of. Issues such as the need to treat early morning surges in blood pressure, the influence of sleep and anxiety disorders on blood pressure, determining the most efficacious first line agent for HTN, therapeutic equivalency of angiotensin converting enzymes and angiotensin receptor blockers, issues and complications in the management of isolated hypertension, and the nature of endothelial dysfunction, among others, receive detailed, focused, and practical treatment in a manner that emphasizes daily application in clinical and hospital settings. Therapeutic approaches emphasize established guidelines for HTN management. Important biochemical and physiologic pathways are illustrated. The emphasis of each chapter is on improving patient care and encouraging clinicians to expand their scope and efficacy of practice.

It is our sincerest wish that this book facilitates the mission each of us share in improving patient care. The targeted, appropriate management of HTN unequivocally reduces cardiovascular morbidity and mortality. The control of HTN also helps to forestall the development of endstage renal disease and need for dialysis and reduces the rate of progression of heart failure, atherosclerosis, and aortic aneurysms. Increasing the number of patients with well-controlled blood pressure is an important goal as it improves the quality and quantity of life. We hope that this book and its companion volume facilitate more aggressive and thoughtful approaches to blood pressure management.

Peter P. Toth
Domenic Sica

1

Do anxiety and panic disorders influence blood pressure?

C. Warren, S. L. Dubovsky

BACKGROUND

The significant comorbidity between hypertension and both generalized and panic anxiety disorders has been recognized for many years [1, 2]. The interaction between anxiety and blood pressure (BP) is complex, involving direct effects of anxiety on BP, lifestyle issues, and effects of psychiatric and antihypertensive medications. In this chapter, we will briefly review the diagnosis and psychiatric comorbidities of anxiety disorders, causes of hypertension in anxious patients, and treatment of anxiety in hypertensive patients.

Anxiety can be broadly divided into generalized, phobic and panic anxiety. Generalized anxiety consists of excessive worry about everyday events. Phobic anxiety is provoked by a particular stimulus or situation. Simple phobias such as fear of snakes or heights are less common than anxiety in social situations (social phobia or social anxiety disorder). Social anxiety may be specific (e.g. anxiety with public speaking or other forms of performance) or it may be generalized (anxiety in all social and performance situations). Panic anxiety is characterized by unprovoked attacks of intense anxiety with substantial physiologic arousal. Recurrent panic attacks are frequently accompanied by anticipatory anxiety (anxiety about having another panic attack) and may lead to agoraphobia, initially manifested as anxiety in any situation in which a panic attack has been experienced or from which escape might be difficult if a panic attack occurred. Agoraphobia may also develop in the absence of panic attacks.

Anxiety disorders are defined by the predominant type of anxiety and the circumstances in which it occurs [3]. For example, generalized anxiety disorder is characterized by chronic, relapsing anxiety involving everyday issues such as worry about something happening to loved ones or about getting sick. Panic disorder is defined by recurrent panic attacks, with or without agoraphobia. Social anxiety disorder and phobias involve anxiety restricted to specific situations or stimuli. Post-traumatic stress disorder is classified with the anxiety disorders, although anxiety is only part of a syndrome of re-experiencing, avoidance, numbing and arousal in response to a severe traumatic event. In obsessive compulsive disorder (OCD), anxiety occurs when patients are not able to engage in compulsions (rituals), which often arise in response to obsessions (for example, when patients with contamination fears

Calvert Warren, MD, Assistant Professor and Director of Psychiatric Emergency Services, Department of Psychiatry, University at Buffalo, Departments of Psychiatry and Medicine, University of Colorado, Buffalo, New York, USA.

Steven L. Dubovsky, MD, Professor and Chair, Department of Psychiatry, University at Buffalo, Departments of Psychiatry and Medicine, University of Colorado, Buffalo, New York, USA.

Table 1.1 Physical symptoms commonly experienced by anxious patients.

- Shortness of breath
- Light headedness
- Paresthesias
- Difficulty concentrating
- Insomnia
- Generalized aches and pains
- Jaw clenching
- Back pain
- Multiple somatic complaints
- Choking
- Chest pain
- Tremor
- Sweating
- Palpitations
- Feeling easily fatigued

are not able to wash their hands after getting them dirty). Anxiety is a prominent secondary symptom in other psychiatric disorders. For example, 70% of depressed patients are also anxious and anxiety can be a symptom of impending overstimulation or mental disorganization in patients with mania or psychosis. Anxiety disorders are most frequently comorbid with other disorders, depression and bipolar disorder; common medical comorbidities include hypertension, dyslipidemias, asthma, and chronic obstructive pulmonary disease [4]. Patients with anxiety and hypertension have an increased rate of non-adherence with medical therapy because they experience more adverse effects and have a lower threshold for discontinuing treatment [2]. Such patients are also less likely to seek medical care in the first place [5].

Psychological dimensions of anxiety involve hyperfocus on the possibility of danger and a sense of being helpless to master it. While mental manifestations of anxiety are obvious (e.g. worry, tension, fears of losing control, difficulty concentrating, avoidance of situations that provoke anxiety), physical symptoms are often the presenting complaint, especially in a non-psychiatric setting (Table 1.1). Physical symptoms represent a combination of exaggerated awareness of minor bodily dysfunction that most people ignore and somatic consequences of high levels of arousal.

PHYSIOLOGY OF ANXIETY

From a physiologic standpoint, anxiety is a state of high arousal. [6, 7]. Arousal in anxiety is mediated by the locus coeruleus, the major brainstem noradrenergic nucleus. Stimulation of the locus coeruleus, can occur with the perception of danger or in response to substances known to induce anxiety such as caffeine, sodium lactate, adrenal medullary hormones, stress, hypotension, hypercapnia or hypoglycemia. Connections to the amygdala result in mental orientation toward the possibility of danger, and activation of the sympathetic nervous system and the hypothalamic-pituitary-adrenal axis results in tremor, tachycardia, elevated BP, altered blood flow, metabolic changes favoring energy production and other dimensions of the 'fight or flight' response.

Whereas anxiety increases central and peripheral release of norepinephrine and its metabolites, catecholamines themselves induce anxiety by activating the locus coeruleus. As a result, stress responses can become self-perpetuating, with the physiology of anxiety leading to more catecholamine release and more arousal. Other stress hormones such as arginine vasopressin, corticotrophin releasing factor and cortisol can also activate the locus coeruleus and induce anxiety. Cholecystokinin also seems to participate in inducing anxiety and may participate in some gastrointestinal symptoms of anxiety.

ASSOCIATION OF ANXIETY AND HYPERTENSION

Anxious patients have an elevated risk of hypertension, and hypertensive patients are more likely than normotensive patients to experience anxiety. In a study of 891 hypertensive outpatients, 11.6% had an anxiety disorder, and levels of anxiety on a self-rating scale were positively correlated with severity and duration of hypertension [8]. State and trait anxiety are both increased in patients with primary hypertension [9]. Similarly, a comparison of 80 hypertensive patients with 80 matched controls reported that anxiety, stress and anger turned inward were more common in hypertensive patients [10], and anxiety and depression but not stress levels were more common in a group of 73 hypertensive patients than in 73 matched controls [11]. A very large Scandinavian population survey found that hypertension was almost twice as common in anxious patients as in controls, while the incidence of hypertension was not increased in patients with schizophrenia [12]. In a retrospective data analysis of 6647 patients with anxiety disorders followed for a year, 22% were hypertensive [4]. A 15-year prospective follow-up of 3308 adults from the Coronary Artery Risk Development in Young Adults (CARDIA) study found that time urgency/impatience and hostility but not anxiety or depression predicted the later development of hypertension [13]; alternatively, in a cross sectional nationally representative telephone and postal survey study of 3032 adults aged 25–74 in the continental US, generalized anxiety disorder in the absence of depression was associated with an increased risk of coronary heart disease [1].

WHAT CAUSES HYPERTENSION IN ANXIOUS PATIENTS?

Anxiety and elevations of BP clearly are associated, but does one cause the other, or are they both consequences of a common factor? Hypertension and anxiety can both result from a number of illnesses and substances [14–17]. A well-known example is pheochromocytoma, which causes both paroxysmal hypertension and anxiety. Hyperthyroidism, hypoglycemia and hypercalcemia are also associated with both anxiety and hypertension. Obesity, which increases the risk of hypertension, is more common in psychiatric disorders, including chronic anxiety disorders [18]. It is not known whether anxious people ingest more salt than the general population, but the average anxious inpatient drinks 20 cups of coffee per day.

Medications such as adrenal steroids, stimulants, sympathomimetics (e.g. phenylephrine), modafinil, progesterone, ergot alkaloids and ropinirole can cause both anxiety and hypertension. Antipsychotic drugs usually cause orthostatic hypotension, but they occasionally elevate BP. These medications also cause akathisia, a sense of inner restlessness, which can make patients markedly anxious. Central nervous system depressants such as the benzodiazepines and barbiturates reduce anxiety acutely, but withdrawal, which frequently occurs between doses of shorter acting medications like alprazolam, causes both anxiety and hypertension, often along with other signs of discontinuation such as tachycardia and tremor. Substances that regularly induce both anxiety and hypertension include caffeine, ephedra, amphetamines and cocaine; tolerance does not develop to the pressor effect of many of these substances, including caffeine [19]. Over-the-counter preparations containing ephedra (banned in the United States since 2004) and caffeine have been reported to cause severe hypertension, sometimes with life-threatening hypertensive encephalopathy [16]. Withdrawal from alcohol induces anxiety, insomnia and hypertension, which may become chronic with ongoing intermittent drinking.

Most antihypertensive medications do not usually cause anxiety, but reserpine, methyldopa, a-adrenergic blocking agents and nifedipine can cause depression, which may then be complicated by anxiety [20]. Beta-adrenergic blocking agents occasionally can cause mania and confusion, which may be accompanied by anxiety. On the other hand, a number of medications commonly used to treat anxiety are associated with hypertension as a side-effect. This is particularly true of medications that increase neurotransmission with dopamine and/ or norepinephrine (e.g. tricyclic antidepressants [TCAs], bupropion, venlafaxine, stimulants) [14]. Venlafaxine can cause severe elevations in BP and hypertensive crises [21]. While they are not directly noradrenergic, the serotonin reuptake inhibitors (SSRIs) indirectly stimulate norepinephrine release, which can then elevate BP. The monoamine oxidase inhibitors (phenelzine, isocarboxazid, tranylcypromine, selegeline), which are used to treat refractory and bipolar depression and some anxiety disorders, interact with tyramine containing foods such as cheese to cause severe hypertension because monoamine oxidase catalyzed degradation of tyramine, a naturally occurring pressor amine, is inhibited by these medications. Occasional cases of spontaneous hypertensive reactions in the absence of dietary indiscretion have been reported with Tranylcypromine. These cases of apparent autoinduction of hypertensive reactions are presumably attributable to metabolic conversion of tranylcypromine to metabolites with pressor activity, although this has not been shown to occur *in vivo*.

Activation of the sympathetic nervous system with anxiety can elevate BP, as was demonstrated by the observation that the prospect of injection of local anesthesia increased systolic and diastolic pressures by 24–26% and 4–5%, respectively [22]. The possibility that anxiety leads directly to hypertension was suggested in a prospective study of 31 healthy men [23]. Over 4.8 years of follow-up, hypertension was significantly more likely to develop in subjects with higher levels of anxiety and irritability and in those with greater BP reactivity in response to stress, but not those with higher salt sensitivity. In a population-based cohort of 3310 initially normotensive healthy individuals followed for up to 22 years, the combination of symptoms of anxiety and depression at baseline are predictive of the risk of later development of hypertension (risk ratio [RR] = 1.73) [24].

A well-known model of the impact of anxiety on BP is the white coat phenomenon (white coat hypertension). In 226 subjects, anxiety in the clinic was significantly associated with higher diastolic BP during clinic visits than at home during ambulatory monitoring [25]. Anxiety during clinic visits is associated with a greater perception of being hypertensive and a larger white coat effect. However, debate continues about the degree to which the white coat phenomenon is a model of clinically important hypertension. In a summary of four prospective cohort studies, white coat hypertension increased the risk of stroke after 9 years of follow-up [26]. In contrast, a 10-year follow-up of 1332 people with either white coat hypertension or hypertension on ambulatory monitoring but not in the doctor's office found that the composite risk of cardiovascular mortality and stroke morbidity was increased in the latter but not the former [27]. This observation seems consistent with other research suggesting that ambulatory monitoring is a better predictor of complications of hypertension than is monitoring in the office, especially by the physician [28].

DOES TREATMENT OF ANXIETY REDUCE BLOOD PRESSURE?

To the extent that anxiety or high levels of arousal contribute to BP elevation, reduction of anxiety should reduce BP. The benzodiazepine diazepam was as effective as sublingual captopril in reducing BP in patients with "excessive" hypertension (BP >190/100 mmHg) referred to an emergency room setting [29]. Thirty years of experience has demonstrated that biofeedback and relaxation therapy can be effective treatments for mild hypertension [30], possibly by attenuating the sympathetic response to stress [31]. In a recent study, a Chinese system of therapy for anxiety resulted in both better BP control and quality of life in hypertensive patients compared with usual care [32]. Controlled studies have demonstrated that transcendental meditation reduces BP, carotid artery intimal thickness, myocardial ischemia, left ventricular hypertrophy and mortality in hypertension [33].

Table 1.2 Some commonly prescribed benzodiazepines.

Drug	Lipid solubility	Half-life	Active metabolites?	Usual daily dose (mg)	Comments
Diazepam	High	Long	Yes	5–30	Rapid onset and offset of action acutely but accumulates over time
Chlordiazepoxide	Low	Long	Yes	25–200	Accumulates with repeated dosing
Clonazepam					
Clorazepate	Low	Short	Yes	7.5–30	Prodrug for desmethyldiazepam
Oxazepam	Low	Short	No	30–60	Useful in liver disease
Lorazepam	Low	Short	No	0.5–2	Slow onset and offset of action in acute dosing
Alprazolam	High	Short	No	0.125–3	Higher doses needed for panic disorder; interdose withdrawal common
Temazepam	Low	Short	No	7.5–30	Usually used as hypnotic but has anxiolytic properties

TREATMENTS FOR ANXIETY IN HYPERTENSIVE PATIENTS

Acute anxiety is usually treated with benzodiazepines [34]. Predictors of a good response include anxiety in response to a specific stress and awareness that symptoms are psychological. These medications all act at benzodiazepine receptors, which allosterically modulate the activity of adjacent gamma-aminobutyric acid (GABA) receptor complexes, organized around a chloride ion channel. Occupation of benzodiazepine receptors increases affinity of GABA receptors for their agonist, increasing chloride influx and hyperpolarizing neurons in limbic, cortical and arousal centers, including the locus coeruleus. Reduction of activity in the locus coeruleus reduces activation of the sympathetic nervous system, with the potential to ameliorate hypertension associated with sympathetic overactivity.

Information about preparations and dosing of benzodiazepines is available in any psychopharmacology text [14]. Table 1.2 categorizes some of the commonly used benzodiazepines according to their lipid solubility and elimination half-life. In general, more lipid soluble medications enter and leave the brain rapidly and therefore have a rapid onset and offset of action after a single dose. If a highly lipid soluble benzodiazepine also has a short elimination half-life, it should be administered more frequently to prevent interdose withdrawal. This problem is most marked with alprazolam, which is also a high potency medication, with rebound of symptoms occurring as the brain level of the medication drops between doses. Medications that are less lipid-soluble have a slower onset of action, and the effect wears off more slowly after a single dose. Benzodiazepines that are relatively low in lipid solubility and have longer elimination half-lives and lower potency (e.g. chlordiazepoxide) accumulate with repeated dosing, resulting in adverse effects beginning some time after starting the medication and persisting for some time after it is discontinued. Diazepam has a long elimination half-life but is highly lipid soluble and it is about five times as potent as chlordiazepoxide. As a result, a single dose works rapidly and the effect wears off quickly, but the medication accumulates with repeated doses. Lorazepam has a relatively short elimination half-life and high potency, but it is low in lipid solubility. Consequently, a single dose has a slower onset and offset of action than a single dose of diazepam, but lorazepam is less likely to accumulate with repeated doses. Oxazepam, an intermediate half-life agent that is the final active metabolite of chlordiazepoxide and diazepam, has no active metabolites of its own. Clorazepate itself has a short half-life but it is a prodrug of desmethyldiazepam with no pharmacologic activity of its own. Its true properties are therefore closer to those of diazepam.

The most important side-effects of the benzodiazepines are sedation and impairment of memory and psychomotor function. The equivalent of 10 mg of diazepam has the potential to impair driving to a degree that would meet criteria for 'driving under the influence'. Tolerance develops to the sedating effects but not the psychomotor impairment that occurs with benzodiazepines. On the other hand, addiction to benzodiazepines is rare in patients who do not have a past history of substance misuse. Discontinuation syndromes, which include return of anxiety, rebound anxiety (anxiety that is more intense than prior to starting the medication), and withdrawal (new physiologic signs such as hypertension, labile BP, tachycardia, myoclonus, confusion and seizures), occur with all benzodiazepines. Drugs with longer half-lives and lower potency (e.g. chlordiazepoxide) are associated with attenuated but more prolonged withdrawal syndromes while benzodiazepines with short half-lives, especially if they are high in potency (e.g. alprazolam) produce more intense withdrawal that appears sooner but does not last as long. Benzodiazepines have additive sedative side-effects with other central nervous system (CNS) depressants and they may have additive hypotensive effects with antihypertensives.

Antidepressants are now the mainstay of treatment of chronic anxiety (Table 1.3). All currently available antidepressants except bupropion are effective for generalized, panic and social anxiety. As was noted earlier, most antidepressants, including the SSRIs, have an initial noradrenergic action that can increase anxiety and BP, in addition to causing related side-effects such as tremor and sweating. However, over time this is followed by down-regulation of β-adrenergic receptors and reduction of noradrenergic activity. Because anxious patients are so sensitive to all adverse effects, antidepressants should be started at a very low dose and the dose should be increased very slowly to allow tolerance to develop to the noradrenergic effect. Beginning treatment with a benzodiazepine can block initial activation by the antidepressant. The benzodiazepine can often be gradually withdrawn when the anxiolytic effect of the antidepressant is fully established. As with the treatment of depression, this can take 1–2 months. Since most anxiety disorders are chronic or recurrent, continuous treatment is often necessary.

The TCAs have been replaced by the SSRIs as first-line treatments because the latter medications have fewer adverse effects and simpler dosing. However, TCAs are still used for more severe and refractory forms of depression as well as for chronic pain and migraine prophylaxis. Anticholinergic side-effects of the TCAs (tachycardia, dry mouth, blurred vision, urinary retention, constipation) are most marked with tertiary amines such as amitriptyline, imipramine, trimipramine and doxepin and less prominent with secondary amines such as desipramine and nortriptyline. Postsynaptic α_1 adrenergic blockade results in hypotension with all TCAs, but noradrenergic TCAs such as desipramine can elevate BP. Alpha-adrenergic blockade also interferes with the pressor action of adrenergic agents such as norepinephrine and dopamine. All of the TCAs have the potential to increase appetite and weight gain, and they all have type 1A antiarrhythmic properties with the potential to aggravate atrioventricular block.

Regardless of manufacturers' claims, all SSRIs have similar efficacy and the same incidence of side-effects, including sexual and gastrointestinal side-effects, headache, sedation and jitteriness. Medications in this class differ in their elimination half-lives and inhibition of CYP450 enzymes. For example, fluoxetine and paroxetine are potent inhibitors of CYP2D6, which metabolizes antihypertensive medications like carvedilol, metoprolol and nebivolol, fluvoxamine inhibits CYP3A4, the isozyme that metabolizes verapamil, diltiazem, and eplerenone.

Table 1.3 Antidepressants.

Drug	Neurotransmitter action	Usual dose (mg)	Blood pressure effects	Comments
Tricyclic antidepressants				
Imipramine	5-HT, NE uptake inhibition	150–300	Postural hypotension	Adjusted by blood level
Desipramine	NE uptake inhibition	150–300	Increased BP	What about the therapeutic window
Amitriptyline	5-HT, NE uptake inhibition	150–300	Postural hypotension	Anticholinergic
Nortriptyline	NE uptake inhibition	75–150	Increased pulse and BP	What about the therapeutic window
Doxepin	NE uptake inhibition; H1 blockade	150–300	Postural hypotension	Useful as antihistamine and for peptic ulcer disease
Trimipramine	NE, 5-HT uptake inhibition	150–300	As for doxepin	
Maprotiline	NE uptake inhibition	150–225	Tetracyclic structure; seizures at doses >225 mg/day	
Amoxapine	NE uptake inhibition, D2 blockade	150–300	Increased BP or postural hypotension	Neuroleptic effect can cause extrapyramidal side-effects; seizures at high doses
Clomipramine	5-HT, NE uptake inhibition	150–250	Postural hypotension	Only TCA effective for OCD
Serotonin reuptake inhibitors				
Fluoxetine		10–40		Half-life 3 days
Paroxetine	5-HT uptake inhibition	10–50		Anticholinergic; causes weight gain; not for use in children
Sertraline		50–200	Negligible	Minimal P450 effects
Fluvoxamine		150–300		Only SSRI to require divided dosing
Citalopram		20–40		No P450 interactions
Escitalopram		10–20		S-enantiomer of citalopram with similar effects
Third-generation antidepressants				
Trazodone	5-HT$_2$, α_1 antagonism	50–600	Hypotension	Can cause priapism at any dose; requires divided dosing as antidepressant
Nefazodone	5-HT$_2$ antagonism, 5-HT uptake inhibition	200–600	Hypotension	Can improve sleep structure; rare cases of severe/fatal hepatotoxicity reported
Bupropion	NE, DA uptake inhibition	150–450	Mild hypertension	No sexual or cardiac effects; seizure risk at doses >450 mg

Table 1.3 Continued.

Drug	Neurotransmitter action	Usual dose (mg)	Blood pressure effects	Comments
SNRIs				
Venlafaxine	5-HT, NE, DA uptake inhibition	75–375	Severe hypertension possible at higher doses	Useful for severe and treatment-resistant depression; divided dose necessary at higher doses of XR formulation
Duloxetine	5-HT, NE uptake inhibition	60–120	Mild hypertension possible	BID dosing
Monoamine oxidase inhibitors				
Phenelzine	Inhibition of intraneural metabolism of 5-HT, NE, DA	30–90	Hypotension; hypertension with dietary interactions	Anticholinergic; causes weight gain
Isocarboxazid	As for phenelzine	20–60	As for phenelzine	Less sedation and weight gain than phenelzine
Tranylcypromine	As for phenelzine; metabolite releases DA	30–90	Less hypotension than phenelzine; spontaneous hypertension possible	More activating; amphetamine-like actions
Selegiline	As for tranylcypromine	20–50	No hypotension; no dietary interactions at doses $\leq$ 10 mg	Minimal antidepressant effect at doses below 20 mg; patch available but benefit may not justify cost

5-HT = serotonin; 5-HT$_2$ = serotonin-2 receptor; BID = twice a day; BP = blood pressure; DA = dopamine; D2 = dopamine 2 receptor; H1 = histamine 1 receptor; HR = heart rate; NE = norepinephrine; OCD = obsessive compulsive disorder; SNRI = serotonin-norepinephrine reuptake inhibitor; SSRI = serotonin reuptake inhibitor; TCA = tricyclic antidepressant; XR = extended release.

Trazodone is primarily an antagonist of serotonin 5-HT$_2$ receptors. Given in doses of 300–600 mg/day on a thrice-daily schedule, trazodone is an antidepressant, but it is too sedating for many patients to tolerate at these high doses. On the other hand, its short elimination half-life makes it useful as a hypnotic. Nefazodone combines SSRI and 5-HT$_2$ antagonist properties. It has negligible effects on BP but occasional cases of severe hepatotoxicity with the proprietary formulation have limited its use. Norepinephrine and to some extent dopamine reuptake inhibition by bupropion carries the potential to increase BP.

Venlafaxine, which is particularly useful for treatment-resistant depression, inhibits serotonin reuptake at doses below 75 mg. As the dose increases, norepinephrine reuptake and then dopamine reuptake are also inhibited. The latter effect produces a risk of significant hypertension in some patients and this medication generally should not be given to hypertensive patients. Duloxetine inhibits reuptake of serotonin and norepinephrine, but not dopamine, at all doses, resulting in a lower risk of hypertension. Mirtazepine antagonizes serotonin 5-HT$_2$ and 5-HT$_3$ receptors as well as presynaptic norepinephrine α_2 receptors, which increases norepinephrine release, with the potential to elevate BP. Venlafaxine, bupropion and mirtazepine therefore are not appropriate initial choices for hypertensive patients.

Monoamine oxidase (MAO) inhibitors are usually prescribed by psychiatrists to treat refractory depression and anxiety disorders. The MAO inhibitor selegiline is also used for Parkinson's disease. Despite their potential to cause dangerous hypertensive reactions when combined with tyramine containing foods and some dopaminergic agents, these medications have a primary hypotensive effect, especially phenelzine and isocarboxazid. Additive hypotensive effects with medications used to treat hypertension are more common than are hypertensive reactions with these compounds.

Buspirone, a 5-HT$_{1A}$ receptor partial agonist, is frequently administered for milder forms of chronic anxiety. As with the antidepressants, buspirone has a slow onset of action. As it does not cause sedation, psychomotor impairment, dependence or withdrawal, it is preferred for patients who cannot tolerate these side-effects (e.g. professional drivers, pilots, patients with pulmonary disease) and for patients with a history of substance abuse. Because of its serotonergic action, buspirone can have dangerous interactions with MAO inhibitors.

The anticonvulsants valproate, gabapentin and pregabalin have been found to have anti-anxiety properties, and gabapentin and pregabalin also have antidepressant effects. These medications are preferable for anxious epileptic patients, and they are second-line treatments for chronic anxiety in patients who should not take or do not respond to the medications listed above. Anticonvulsants do not have predictable BP effects,

A few antihypertensive medications are also used to treat certain anxiety disorders such as 10–20 mg of propranolol being used acutely for performance anxiety. Prazosin has recently been shown to decrease nightmares and agitation in patients with post-traumatic stress disorder [35], although it does not treat other symptoms of this condition. Clonidine is occasionally used to treat severe anxiety, but it is more frequently used to reduce the hyperactivity in attention deficit disorder.

Behavioral therapies such as relaxation, biofeedback, meditation and hypnosis should be considered for all chronically anxious patients. These therapies not only are effective in their own right, but they increase patients' active involvement in treatment, creating a sense of mastery that counteracts the feelings of helplessness that are intrinsic to anxiety. In contrast, waiting for a pill to start working without a sense of personal engagement can intensify feelings of passivity. Since behavioral therapies can also ameliorate hypertension, they may reduce the total amount of medication that is needed.

SUMMARY

Anxiety disorders are common conditions that frequently coexist with hypertension. The physiology of anxiety can contribute to moderate hypertension but by itself it is probably not sufficient to cause persistent severe elevations of BP. Clinicians treating anxious patients should consider medical causes and side-effects of medications and non-prescription substances before adding anti-anxiety medications. Acute anxiety is generally treated by addressing the cause of the anxiety and as necessary with the addition of a benzodiazepine. Anticonvulsants may be useful anxiolytics for patients with a history of substance abuse. When antidepressants and buspirone are used in the treatment of anxiety their delayed onset of action should be taken into account.

Behavioral therapies should be considered for all chronically anxious patients. Treatment of anxiety often improves BP control but by itself is not likely to be fully effective when more severe hypertension is present. Anxious patients are less likely than other patients to seek treatment for hypertension in the first place, and when they do they are more likely to discontinue treatment prematurely because of high sensitivity to side-effects.

REFERENCES

1. Barger SD, Sydeman SJ. Does generalized anxiety disorder predict coronary heart disease risk factors independently of major depressive disorder? *J Affect Disord* 2005; 88:87–91.
2. Davies SJC, Jackson PR, Ramsay LE, Ghahramani P. Drug intolerance due to nonspecific adverse effects related to psychiatric morbidity in hypertensive patients. *Arch Intern Med* 2003; 163:592–600.
3. Association AP. *Diagnostic and Statistical Manual of Mental Disorders,* 4th edition. American Psychiatric Press, Washington, D.C., 1994.
4. McLaughlin T, Geissler EC, Wan GJ. Comorbidities and associated treatment charges in patients with anxiety disorders. *Pharmacotherapy* 2003; 23:1251–1256.
5. Cradock-O'Leary J, Young AS, Yano EM, Wang M, Lee ML. Use of general medical services by VA patients with psychiatric disorders. *Psychiatr Serv* 2002; 53:874–878.
6. Roman O, Seres J, Pometlova M, Jurcovicora J. Neuroendocrine or behavioral effects of acute or chronic emotional stress in Wistar Kyoto (WKY) and spontaneously hypertensive (SHR) rats. *Endocr Regul* 2004; 38:151–155.
7. Dubovsky SL, Dubovsky AN. *Concise Guide to Mood Disorders.* American Psychiatric Press, Washington, D.C., 2002.
8. Wei TM, Wang L. Anxiety symptoms in patients with hypertension: a community-based study. *Int J Psychiatry Med* 2006; 36:315–322.
9. Nasilowska-Barud A, Kowalik M. Characteristics of depressive changes and anxiety in patients with essential hypertension. *Ann Univ Mariae Curie Sklodowska Med* 2004; 59:428–433.
10. Sharma S. Life events stress, emotional vital signs and hypertension. *Psychol Stud (Mysore)* 2003; 48:53–65.
11. Frances F, Calvo PD, Diaz OB, Ramal J, Aleman S. Differences in anxiety, depression, stress and social support between hypertensive and normotensive subjects. *Ansiedad y Estres* 2001; 7:203–213.
12. Johannessen L, Strudsholm U, Foldager L, Munk-Jorgensen P. Increased risk of hypertension in patients with bipolar disorder and patients with anxiety compared to background population and patients with schizophrenia. *J Affect Disord* 2006; 95:13–17.
13. Yan LL, Liu K, Matthews KA, Daviglus ML, Ferguson TF, Kiefe CI. Psychosocial factors and risk of hypertension: The Coronary Artery Risk Development in Young Adults (CARDIA) Study. JAMA 2003; 290:2138–2148.
14. Dubovsky SL. *Clinical Guide to Psychotropic Medications.* WW Norton, New York, 2005.
15. Walsh JP, Bremner AP, Bulsara MK *et al.* Subclinical thyroid dysfunction and blood pressure: a community-based study. *Clin Endocrinol (Oxf)* 2006; 65:486–491.
16. Berman JA, Setty A, Steiner MJ, Kaufman KR, Skotzko C. Complicated hypertension related to the abuse of ephedrine and caffeine alkaloids. *J Addict Dis* 2006; 25:45–48.
17. Coleman JJ, Martin U. Drug-induced systemic hypertension. *Adverse Drug React Bull* 2006; 239:915–918.
18. Susce MT, Villanueva N, Diaz FJ, de Leon J. Obesity and associated complications in patients with severe mental illnesses: a cross-sectional survey. *J Clin Psychiatry* 2005; 66:167–173.
19. James JE. Critical review of dietary caffeine and blood pressure: a relationship that should be taken more seriously. *Psychosom Med* 2004; 66:63–71.

20. Hullett FJ, Potkin SG, Levy AB, Ciasca R. Depression associated with nifedipine-induced calcium channel blockers. *Am J Psychiatry* 1988; 145:1277–1279.

21. Khurana RN, Baudendistel TE. Hypertensive crisis associated with venlafaxine. *Am J Med* 2003; 115:676–677.

22. van den Berg AA. Bradycardia and hypertension in anticipation of, and exacerbated by, peribulbar block: a prospective audit. *Acta Anaesthesiol Scand* 2005; 49:1207–1213.

23. Deter HC, Micus C, Wagner M, Sharma AM, Bucholz K. Salt sensitivity, anxiety, and irritability predict blood pressure increase over five years in healthy males. *Clin Exp Hypertens* 2006; 28:17–27.

24. Jonas BS, Lando JF. Negative affect as a prospective risk factor for hypertension. *Psychosom Med* 2000; 62:188–196.

25. Jhalani J, Goyal T, Clemow L, Schwartz JE, Pickering TG, Gerin W. Anxiety and outcome expectations predict the white-coat effect. *Blood Press Monit* 2005; 10:317–319.

26. Angeli F, Verdecchia P, Gattobigio R, Sardone M, Reboldi G. White coat hypertension in adults. *Blood Press Monit* 2005; 10:301–305.

27. Ohkubo T, Kikuya M, Metoki H *et al.* Prognosis of "masked" hypertension and "white-coat" hypertension detected by 24-h ambulatory blood pressure monitoring: 10-year follow-up from the Ohasama study. *J Am Coll Cardiol* 2005; 46:508–515.

28. Stergiou GS, Kalogeropoulos PG, Baibas NM. Prognostic value of home blood pressure measurement. *Blood Press Monit* 2007; 12:391–392.

29. Grossman E, Nadler M, Sharabi Y, Thaler M, Shachar A, Shamiss A. Antianxiety treatment in patients with excessive hypertension. *Am J Hypertens* 2005; 18:1174–1177.

30. Richter-Heinrich E, Knust U, Lori M, Sprung H. Control of blood pressure during biofeedback in patients with essential hypertension. *Z Psychol Z Angew Psychol* 1976; 184:538–550.

31. Tsai PS, Chang NC, Chang WY, Lee PH, Wang MY. Blood pressure biofeedback exerts intermediate-term effects on blood pressure and pressure reactivity in individuals with mild hypertension: a randomized controlled study. *J Altern Complement Med* 2007; 13:547–554.

32. Duan S, Xiao J, Zhao S-p, Zhu X-z. The effect of antianxiety on the blood pressure and life quality of hypertension patients with anxiety. *Chin J Clin Psychol* 2008; 16:205–207.

33. Walton KS, Schneider RH, Nidich SI, Salerno JW, Nordstrom CK, Bairey Merz CN. Psychosocial stress and cardiovascular disease Part 2: effectiveness of the Transcendental Meditation program in treatment and prevention. *Behav Med* 2002; 28:106–123.

34. Dubovsky SL. Agents acting on the benzodiazepine receptor. In: Sadock B, Sadock V, Ruiz P (eds). *Comprehensive Textbook of Psychiatry IX*. Williams and Wilkins, Baltimore, 2009.

35. Taylor FB, Martin P, Thompson C *et al.* Prazosin effects on objective sleep measures and clinical symptoms in civilian post-traumatic stress disorder: a placebo-controlled study. *Biol Psychiatry* 2008; 63:629–632.

2

Should diuretic therapy be first step therapy in all hypertensive patients?

B. L. Carter, M. E. Ernst

BACKGROUND

One of the most contentious issues currently surrounding the treatment of hypertension involves the role of diuretics. These agents have been available for 50 years but their optimal use and place in therapy continue to be actively debated [1–3]. Over 70 million people suffer from hypertension in the United States while only 37% have achieved goal blood pressure [4]. This chapter will focus on thiazides (e.g. hydrochlorothiazide [HCTZ]) and thiazide-like (chlorthalidone) diuretics that are the primary agents demonstrating efficacy in reducing morbidity and mortality in hypertensive patients. We will refer to both HCTZ and chlorthalidone as thiazide diuretics in this chapter and focus on essential hypertension. Loop or high-ceiling diuretics, which are more useful in renal failure and volume overload conditions, will not be discussed.

Even experts who often disagree on when diuretics should be used are in agreement on several important principles relating to hypertension therapy [2, 3]. These principles include the following:

- The most important goal is to control the blood pressure to targets recommended in guidelines [5].
- Most patients require an average of 2–3 antihypertensive medications to achieve blood pressure goals [6, 7].
- A common cause of suspected resistant hypertension is the lack of a suitably dosed diuretic in the regimen [8].
- Diuretics have been found to be superior to angiotensin converting enzyme (ACE) inhibitors, α-blockers and calcium channel blockers (CCBs) in their ability to significantly reduce the development of heart failure (HF) in patients with hypertension [2, 3, 9, 10].

The Antihypertensive and Lipid-Lowering Treatment to Prevent Heart Attack Trial (ALLHAT) [6], network meta-analyses [11], and the Seventh Report of the Joint National Committee on Prevention, Detection, Evaluation and Treatment of High Blood Pressure

Barry L. Carter, PharmD, FCCP, FAHA, Professor, Department of Pharmacy Practice and Science, College of Pharmacy and Department of Family Medicine, College of Medicine, University of Iowa, Iowa City, Iowa, USA.

Michael E. Ernst, PharmD, FCCP, Professor (Clinical), Department of Pharmacy Practice and Science, College of Pharmacy and Department of Family Medicine, College of Medicine, University of Iowa, Iowa City, Iowa, USA.

(JNC-7) [5] all suggest that diuretics should be first-line therapy for hypertension. Even so, only about 26% of antihypertensive regimens in the US include a thiazide-type diuretic [12, 13]. The failure to include a thiazide diuretic in many therapeutic regimens contributes to the large number of patients with poorly controlled BP.

This chapter will review the controversy surrounding the use of thiazide diuretics as first-step therapy for hypertension. We will attempt to provide a balanced view on this topic. We will also discuss whether all diuretics should be considered equivalent for the treatment of hypertension. In addition, we will address other important and controversial issues such as thiazide-induced new onset diabetes mellitus.

IMPORTANT QUESTIONS

WHAT HAS BEEN THE EVOLUTION OF THE STEPPED-CARE CONCEPT AS PER THE JNC GUIDE-LINES?

The earliest versions of the JNC guidelines used the stepped-care approach to the pharmacologic treatment of hypertension. The principle at play was to initiate therapy with a thiazide diuretic at a moderate dose and thereafter to titrate to a maximal effective dose. If BP was not controlled, a second-line drug was added and it also titrated to moderate or maximal dosages. This process continued until the patient was taking three or four medications as necessary. It should be noted that in the early 1970s when the stepped-care approach emerged, there were only a handful of non-diuretic medications available for the treatment of hypertension including alpha methyldopa, hydralazine and reserpine. Since these non-diuretic agents often caused dose-dependent fluid retention, it was frequently necessary to have a diuretic in the regimen if treatment resistance was to be avoided. It is also important to realize that dose ranging in the early years of diuretic use involved daily doses of up to 200 and 100 mg, respectively for HCTZ and chlorthalidone. These high diuretic doses offered little incremental benefit for BP reduction (compared to lower doses) and often produced troubling dose-dependent adverse metabolic effects [1, 14, 15]. Minor modifications in this stepped-care approach continued through the mid-1980s.

When the JNC IV guidelines were published in 1988, β-blockers, CCBs and ACE inhibitors had been available for several years. Not unsurprisingly, the JNC IV guidelines incorporated these newer drug classes into therapy recommendations now suggesting that either a diuretic, β-blocker, CCB or ACE inhibitor would be suitable first-step therapies (in addition to non-pharmacologic therapy) [16]. These recommendations regarding first-step status for non-diuretic therapies were made despite the absence of definitive outcomes trials with β-blockers, CCBs or ACE inhibitors.

A more evidence-based approach, than was the case for previous reports, was taken with the JNC-V guidelines but nonetheless the final document still remained a consensus-driven process [17]. Diuretics or β-blockers were preferred as first-line therapy in JNC-V in that these were the only two drug classes having been shown to reduce morbidity and mortality. These guidelines deviated somewhat from the old 'stepped' approach in suggesting three options if there was an inadequate response to the initial drug chosen. These options were to:

1. Increase the dose of the first drug;
2. Substitute a medication from a different drug class; or
3. Add a second drug from a different pharmacologic class.

This JNC-V report was immediately criticized on several fronts, being described in an accompanying editorial as *"hypertension: steps forward and steps backward"* [18]. The authors of this editorial were critical of the fact that JNC-V relied too heavily on the results of the Systolic Hypertension in the Elderly (SHEP) trial and argued that CCBs and ACE

Table 2.1 Pharmacokinetics and pharmacodynamic comparisons of hydrochlorothiazide and chlorthalidone (adapted with permission from [1, 25]).

Drug	Onset (hours)	Peak (hours)	Half-life (hours)	Duration (hours)
Hydrochlorothiazide	2	4–6	6–9 (single dose) 8–15 (chronic dosing)	8–12 (single dose) 12–16 (chronic dosing)
Chlorthalidone	2–3	2–6	40 (single dose) 45–60 (chronic dosing)	24–48 (single dose) 48–72 (chronic dosing)

inhibitors had proven vascular effects that could be extrapolated to a presumed benefit on morbidity and mortality (which should be noted would not have been in any way evidence-based).

Even stronger evidence-based approaches were taken with JNC-VI and 7. Diuretics and β-blockers continued to be recommended as first-line therapy in JNC-VI [19]. JNC-7 suggested that diuretics should be considered as the preferred first-line agents primarily based on the results of the ALLHAT trial [6]. JNC-7 removed β-blockers as first-line therapy in uncomplicated hypertension based on the findings from several reports suggesting that β-blockers, primarily atenolol, did not provide the reductions in cardiovascular (CV) events expected with a BP-reducing compound [2, 3].

At the time of this writing, the JNC-8 panel has been assembled but the report is not anticipated until 2011. The JNC-8 is taking an even stronger evidence-based approach and will be structured in a similar manner to other evidence-based guidelines committees, which define key questions and provide levels or strengths of evidence to support the recommendations offered.

ARE ALL DIURETICS TO BE CONSIDERED AS BEING EQUAL IN THE TREATMENT OF HYPERTENSION?

Before clinical trials can be appropriately evaluated, the issue of whether all thiazide diuretics should be considered equal must first be addressed. To answer this question, several key points must be noted. First, the only diuretics shown to reduce morbidity and mortality in hypertension are thiazide diuretics, including the thiazide-like diuretic chlorthalidone [2]. Second, the majority of scientific evidence on the favorable effects of diuretic therapy has been generated with HCTZ and chlorthalidone. Therefore, we will focus on those two agents. The Hypertension in the Very Elderly Trial (HYVET) study used a sustained-release form of indapamide as initial therapy and that study will be briefly discussed [20].

All of the recent JNC documents generally considered the thiazides, especially HCTZ and chlorthalidone, as being interchangeable. These guidelines also suggested that low doses (12.5–50 mg) of HCTZ and chlorthalidone were therapeutically equivalent. In addition, current versions of authoritative pharmacology textbooks, such as Goodman and Gilman's, list the diuretic potency as 1:1 for these two agents [21]. This 1:1 equivalence issue, however, was not borne out by available outcomes data in that chlorthalidone seemed to provide greater improvements in morbidity and mortality than studies that used HCTZ. This between drug difference for outcomes could have related to antihypertensive efficacy differences and/or pharmacokinetic distinctions between these two compounds [1, 22]. For example, chlorthalidone has a much longer duration of action than HCTZ and is nearly twice as potent as HCTZ (Table 2.1) [1]. Chlorthalidone is unique because it heavily compartmentalizes into red blood cells by binding to carbonic anhydrase and then slowly 'back leaks' into serum [23, 24].This backleaking into serum occurs such that a constant equilibrium exists between the amount of drug bound to carbonic anhydrase in the red blood cell compartment and the amount of free drug available in the plasma compartment. This depot effect is the basis for the extended diuretic (and presumably antihypertensive) actions of chlorthalidone [23, 24].

The comparative antihypertensive effects of "equivalent" doses of chlorthalidone and HCTZ has only recently been examined. Ernst and colleagues compared 50 mg of HCTZ to 25 mg of chlorthalidone in how each influenced both office and 24-h ambulatory BP values. In spite of similar reductions in clinic BP, 24-h monitoring revealed a significantly lower night time BP with chlorthalidone at half the dose of hydrochlorothiazide [25].

What message can be derived from these data? First, BP lowering and achieving goal BP remains the most important principle. In this regard, monotherapy with chlorthalidone is more effective than HCTZ, especially at lowering BP throughout the entire 24-h treatment interval. These data do not imply that HCTZ is a poor antihypertensive *per se* or that it is necessarily inferior to chlorthalidone when used in an appropriate combination regimen. In addition, outcome studies, which favored HCTZ-based therapy over non-diuretic agents used higher doses and often used the drug twice daily. Therefore, doses of chlorthalidone should be 12.5–25 mg *once daily* while the appropriate evidence-based dose for hydrochlorothiazide to achieve similar BP control is likely 12.5–25 mg *twice daily*. These are significant differences in dosage that must be considered before appropriate interpretations of the clinical trials comparing thiazides with other classes can be made. At these doses, the metabolic effects, especially hypokalemia, are similar between these two diuretics [15, 25].

SHOULD WE BE CONCERNED ABOUT NEW ONSET DIABETES MELLITUS ATTRIBUTED TO THIAZIDE DIURETICS?

One of the concerns among clinicians that may contribute to the avoidance of thiazide therapy is the development of new onset diabetes mellitus (DM) following their initiation. Many authors continue to discourage thiazides as initial therapy for uncomplicated hypertension because of this (and other) metabolic effects (although they are recommended for patients at higher risk) [3, 26]. What has largely been underappreciated until recently is that there appears be a relationship between thiazide-induced hyperglycemia and hypokalemia, a relationship, interestingly enough, that has been well described since the 1950s [27, 28].

Studies have consistently found increased serum glucose levels following the use of thiazide diuretics [6, 28–33]. In ALLHAT, most of the patients who developed new onset DM had a small increase in serum glucose (3–4 mg/dl), but because incident DM was defined in a dichotomous manner (fasting blood sugar >126-mg/dl), a significantly higher number of 'new diabetics' were found in the thiazide-treated group. Diuretic-induced hyperglycemia is the portion of the increase in serum glucose levels that is above the increase related to aging, weight gain, sedentary life style, and other risk factors [33]. This distinction is important because 83% of the new onset DM that occurred in the ALLHAT diuretic arm was likely not due to diuretic therapy as glucose was found to increase in treated groups regardless of their antihypertensive regimen [6, 34].

While the evidence is somewhat contradictory, in most instances there is a slight increase in absolute risk for new onset DM following thiazide use. Elliott and Meyer published a meta-analysis of 22 clinical trials involving 143 153 participants and found that placebo groups had a significantly lower odds ratio (OR) of developing DM (OR 0.77; confidence interval [CI] 0.63–0.94) when compared to those who received thiazides [35]. The odds ratio for CCBs (OR 0.75; CI 0.62–0.90), ACE inhibitors (OR 0.67; CI 0.56–0.80) and angiotensin II receptor blockers (ARBs) (OR 0.57; CI 0.46–0.72) were also significantly reduced compared to thiazide treated patients.

An important point about thiazide-induced DM is that the ALLHAT as well as long-term follow-up from the Systolic Hypertension in the Elderly Program study have not yet found detrimental effects from new onset DM [6, 36]. Diuretic-based therapy in ALLHAT resulted in similar or superior major CV benefits compared to lisinopril or amlodipine, even in patients with DM and in those with the metabolic syndrome [37–40]. This finding is not surprising considering that adverse risk with glucose is a continuous relationship and small changes, as were seen in ALLHAT, likely impart a small risk. In fact, if being labeled a diabetic prompts further aggressive measures to control BP and other CV risk factors, it may be a serendipitous finding. However, it has also been argued that the length of follow-up in clinical trials was only 2–5 years, which was too short to recognize any long-term adverse effects from new onset DM [26]. One small study suggested that new onset DM carried the same CV risk as DM when present prior to therapy [26]. Regardless, any new cases of thiazide-induced diabetes are a concern because they require additional monitoring and treatment and these patients could likely have increased risk over many years or decades. Therefore, strategies to limit new onset diabetes with thiazides are important. This controversy has created a great deal of "noise", which has caused many physicians to avoid thiazides leading to suboptimal control of hypertension. This failure to control hypertension is believed to result in more cases of heart failure, myocardial infarction and strokes. Even so, if thiazide-induced diabetes could be prevented, it would greatly improve the management of hypertension and the acceptance of thiazides. Because it appears that hypokalemia may be a contributing factor to the development of new onset DM, it is important to prevent hypokalemia, although it is not clear to what degree thiazide-induced diabetes is forestalled by this [28, 41].

A meta-analysis of 59 studies involving thiazides was recently undertaken. Trial size, trial length, and type/dosage of thiazide diuretic varied substantially among the studies. The most commonly used thiazides were chlorthalidone and HCTZ with total daily doses ranging from 12.5 to 100 mg per day for chlorthalidone and from 12.5 to 400 mg per day for HCTZ. A significant correlation between the degree of diuretic-induced hypokalemia and an increase in plasma glucose was observed [28]. These results suggest that prevention of hypokalemia with potassium supplementation or potassium-sparing agents could reduce the level of hyperglycemia following diuretic therapy [28]. It is likely that there are multiple mechanisms that contribute to the development of thiazide-induced diabetes including stimulation of the sympathetic nervous system and the renin-angiotensin-aldosterone system; however, the exact relationship between level of activation of these neurohumoral pathways and degree of hyperglycemia is not well understood [33].

If hyperglycemia or DM develops with the use of thiazides, it is important to recognize that, absent changes in serum potassium, many of these cases are not related to the thiazide itself. The lifestyle factors that increased the risk for diabetes will likely lead to future DM even if the thiazide is stopped. This is an important observation in that a thiazide diuretic will usually be necessary to achieve tight BP control in the diabetic patient with hypertension. The evidence shows that CV risk reduction following thiazide use extends to those who develop DM on treatment. We believe that because the overwhelming evidence supports lowering of CV events with lowering of BP, while the evidence of harm from impairments in glucose metabolism or increased insulin resistance due to diuretics is not firmly established, that an argument could be made that it is ill-advised, if not unethical, to withhold a thiazide diuretic in the setting of DM when hypertension remains uncontrolled.

The lowest thiazide dose should be selected when diuretic therapy is being initiated (chlorthalidone 6.25–12.5 mg *once daily* or hydrochlorothiazide 12.5 mg *twice daily*). Hydrochlorothiazide once daily can only be justified when it is used in combination with other drugs with clear 24-h durations of action. Most importantly, in the patient with hypertension, BP must be controlled (<130/80 mmHg in the patient with diabetes and/or chronic kidney disease) and some patients will require up titration to chlorthalidone 25 mg *once daily* or HCTZ 25 mg *twice daily* to achieve their goal. While there may be some modest reduction in BP if higher doses are used, we do not believe higher doses can be justified in most patients due to the increasing risk of metabolic adverse effects. We suggest chlorthalidone (at these doses) as a preferred option because it achieves better 24-h BP control with no increase in hypokalemia when compared to HCTZ [25]. In addition, we do not favor the inconvenience of dosing a diuretic in the evening due to the potential for nocturia. Patients should also be advised to adhere to a low salt, high potassium diet as hypokalemia due to thiazides is worsened by high dietary sodium intake. There are many foods high in potassium such as fruits, vegetables and now many low sodium foods. However, it is often difficult to reverse hypokalemia without other measures such as sodium restriction, potassium supplementation or a potassium-sparing diuretic. Our recent meta-analysis found an average reduction in serum K^+ of 0.23 mmol/l and an increase in glucose of but 3.26 mg/dl in studies using potassium supplements or potassium-sparing agents. In studies that did not use these agents, the average reduction in serum potassium was 0.37 mmol/l, with an average increase in serum glucose of 6.01 mg/dl ($P = 0.03$). The lowest rates of CV risk and glucose intolerance appear to occur at serum K^+ values between 4.0 and 4.5 mmol/l [28, 42]. Potassium supplements or potassium-sparing agents should be added if baseline serum potassium values are below 4.0 mmol/l or if it falls below this level during therapy; however, it is still debated whether all patients taking a diuretic should be maintained at a serum potassium value greater than 4.0-mmol/l. With hypokalemia and uncontrolled hypertension, our approach is to suggest either amiloride or low-dose spironolactone, which are both very effective in patients with resistant hypertension and they are more effective at increasing serum potassium than is the case for oral potassium [33, 43, 44]. Antihypertensive regimens can also be designed so as to minimize hypokalemia and, hopefully, hyperglycemia. For instance, the addition of an angiotension converting enzyme (ACE) inhibitor can minimize or negate the effects of thiazide's capacity to cause electrolyte disturbances such as hypokalemia, as well as to variably effect diuretic-related hyperlipidemia and glucose intolerance [45, 46]. The same positive effects on glucose homeostasis should be expected with angiotensin receptor blockers therapy; however, this did not occur with losartan/HCTZ (50–100/12.5–25-mg/day) in the Study of Trandolapril/Verapamil SR And insulin Resistance (STAR) [47].

WHAT ARE THE RESULTS FROM OUTCOME STUDIES COMPARING DIURETICS TO OTHER DRUG CLASSES?

The reason guideline committees in the US have suggested that thiazide-type diuretics are preferred as initial therapy is based on over four decades of positive clinical trial results, including active-controlled trials where diuretics were tested against other drugs for their efficacy in preventing hard clinical outcomes such as myocardial infarction, death, stroke, HF and renal failure. Table 2.2 summarizes many of the critical studies that have been conducted with thiazide-based therapy. Several different thiazide-type diuretics and/or β-blockers in combination with diuretics have been studied as initial therapy; however, results have not been routinely separated by type of diuretic or other concomitant therapies (e.g. potassium-sparing agents) [48–53].

Some studies included only elderly subjects (e.g. SHEP, European Working Party Trial, Medical Research Council trial). Others, such as the ALLHAT, over-sampled African Americans while the Second Australian National Blood Pressure Study (ANBP2) included very few blacks. It is intriguing to note that of the several trials reporting neutral or negative results in the diuretic groups that HCTZ was used [54–58], while those with more favorable outcomes utilized chlorthalidone [6, 22, 59–62]. The studies with favorable outcomes with HCTZ often used doses of 50 mg daily or more and frequently administered HCTZ twice daily.

One of the major exceptions to the belief that conventional dose HCTZ offers limited outcomes benefits was the Hypertension in the Very Elderly Trial (HYVET) [20]. This was a randomized, double-blind, placebo-controlled study that compared sustained release indapamide (1.5 mg) with or without perindopril (2–4 mg) to placebo in 3845 patients over the age of 80 years. The target BP in this study was <150/80 mmHg. At two years there was a 21% reduction in all-cause death (95% CI 4–35; $P = 0.02$), a 39% reduction in fatal stroke (95%

Table 2.2 Clinical trials using hydrochlorothiazide or chlorthalidone-based therapy (adapted with permission from [15, 24]).

Trial (Year Published)	Regimen*	Population	Outcome
Clinical trials with HCTZ-based regimens			
Oslo Hypertension Study (1982) [56]	HCTZ 50 mg/day (36%), HCTZ 50 mg/day + propranolol 320 mg/day (26%), HCTZ 50 mg/day + methyldopa 1000 mg/day (20%), or other drugs (18%) compared to no treatment	Men aged 40–49 years (406 treated and 379 untreated); BP (baseline): 156/97 mmHg; 17/10 mmHg reduction (SDP/DBP) vs. untreated	More non-coronary events in untreated (P <0.001); more coronary events in treated (14) compared to untreated (3), (P <0.01)
European Working Party on High Blood Pressure in the Elderly (EWPHBPE) (1985) [66]	HCTZ 25–50 mg + triamterene 50–100 mg; methyldopa 500–2000 mg could be added, compared to placebo	840 patients over 60 years BP (baseline): 183/101 mmHg BP (active treatment): 148/85 mmHg BP (placebo): 167/90 mmHg	CV mortality reduced 27% (P = 0.037), cardiac mortality 38% (P = 0.036) in active treatment group; no change in total mortality (P = 0.41)
Metoprolol Atherosclerosis Prevention in Hypertensives (MAPHY) (1988) [57]	Metoprolol vs. HCTZ 50 mg daily or bendroflumethiazide 5 mg daily	1609 men aged 40–64 years BP (baseline): 167/107 mmHg BP (treatment): 142/89 mmHg	Metoprolol treated subjects had significantly lower CV mortality (P = 0.012), CHD mortality (P = 0.048), stroke mortality (P = 0.043) or total mortality (P = 0.28) compared to diuretics
Medical Research Council (MRC) (1992) [55]	HCTZ 25–50 mg + amiloride 2.5–5 mg vs. Atenolol 50 mg vs. Placebo	4396 patients 65–74 years BP (baseline): 185/91 mmHg BP (diuretic): 150/78 mmHg BP (atenolol): 152/78 mmHg	31% fewer strokes (P = 0.04) in HCTZ group, 44% fewer coronary events (P = 0.0009) and 35% fewer CV events (P = 0.0005) compared to placebo. No significant reductions in outcomes for atenolol group.
Multicenter Isradipine Diuretic Atherosclerosis Study (MIDAS) (1996) [67]	HCTZ 12.5–25 mg BID vs. Isradipine 2.5–5 mg BID; open label enalapril could be added	883 patients; mean age = 58 years. BP with HCTZ decreased from 149/96 mmHg to 130/82 mmHg; BP with isradipine decreased from 151/97 mmHg to 135/84 mmHg	Fewer major vascular events (3.2% vs. 5.7%, P = 0.07) and fewer non-major vascular events (5.2% vs. 9.1%, P = 0.02) with HCTZ than isradipine
International Nifedipine GITS Study (INSIGHT) (2000) [68]	HCTZ 25–50 mg + amiloride 50–100 mg vs. nifedipine GITS 30–60 mg and atenolol or enalapril could be added	6321 patients aged 55–80 years; Similar BP decline in both groups from 173/99 mmHg to 138/82 mmHg	No difference overall in combined (primary and secondary) endpoints. However, there were more fatal MIs (16 vs. 5; OR 3.2, P = 0.017) and non-fatal heart failure (24 vs. 11; OR 2.2; P = 0.028) with nifedipine compared to the diuretic

Table 2.2 Continued.

Trial (Year Published)	Regimen*	Population	Outcome
Second Australian National Blood Pressure Study (ANBP-2) (2003) [54]	Randomized to either HCTZ or enalapril (doses were adjusted by family practitioner and not reported)	6083 patients aged 65–84 years: BP (baseline) 168/91 mmHg; BP (HCTZ): 144/81 mmHg; BP (enalapril): 145/81 mmHg	Significantly fewer CV events or deaths in enalapril group compared to HCTZ (HR = 0.89; P = 0.05).
Avoiding Cardiovascular Events through Combination Therapy in Patients Living with Systolic Hypertension (ACCOMPLISH) (2008) [58]	Randomized to amlodipine 5–10 mg + benazepril 20–40 mg OR benazepril 20–40 mg + HCTZ 12.5–25 mg.	11 462 patients ≥55 years, SBP ≥160 mmHg	RR 0.8 (0.72–0.90) for composite of CV mortality/morbidity for amlodipine-benazepril group vs. benazepril-HCTZ group (P = 0.0002)
Trials with chlorthalidone-based regimens			
Hypertension Detection and Follow-up Program (HDFP) (1979) [59]	Stepped care (SC) using chlorthalidone as Step 1 compared to regular care (RC) consisting of multiple regimens and doses	10 940 patients age 30–69 years; BP (baseline): 159/101 mmHg; Reported DBP only: RC 89 mmHg; SC 84 mmHg	17% lower mortality in SC than RC groups (P < 0.01). Total stroke was lower in the SC than RC groups (P <0.01)
Multiple Risk Factor Intervention Trial (MRFIT) (1990) [22]	Randomized to special intervention (SI) or usual care (UC). Step 1 included either HCTZ or chlorthalidone (50–100 mg daily). Mid-study protocol changed HCTZ to chlorthalidone	8012 hypertensive men; BP (baseline): 141/91 mmHg; BP (UC group): 130/86 mmHg; BP (SI group): 122/81 mmHg	Mortality reduced 36% (P = 0.07) and CHD reduced 50% (P = 0.0001) in SI group vs. UC. Early mortality was 44% higher in SI clinics using HCTZ vs. UC but was 28% lower following a change from HCTZ to chlorthalidone (P = 0.04 comparing the two time periods)
Systolic Hypertension in the Elderly (SHEP) (1991) [61]	Randomized to chlorthalidone 12.5–25 mg and could add atenolol 25 mg or reserpine 0.05 mg vs. placebo	4736 patients, mean age 72 years BP (baseline): 170/76 mmHg; BP (chlorthalidone): 144/68 mmHg; BP (placebo): 155/71 mmHg	Significant reduction in stroke for chlorthalidone compared to placebo (RR = 0.64; P = 0.0003); 32% fewer combined non-fatal and fatal CV events in chlorthalidone group. Heart failure reduced 54% in chlorthalidone group compared to placebo.

Treatment of Mild Hypertension Study (TOMHS) (1993) [69]	Randomized to chlorthalidone 15–30 mg/day (136 patients), acebutolol 400 mg/day (132 patients), doxazosin 1–2 mg/day (134 patients), amlodipine 5 mg/day (131 patients), or enalapril 5 mg/day (135 patients) vs. placebo; chlorthalidone could be added to placebo if nutritional-hygienic intervention did not control BP	Men and women 45 to 69 years of age; BP (baseline): 140/91 mmHg; largest reduction in systolic BP in chlorthalidone group (-17.7 mmHg)	Rate of all clinical events was 11.1% in combined active treatments vs. 16.2% for placebo ($P = 0.03$); no consistent differences among active treatments for LV mass, lipid levels or other outcomes
Antihypertensive and Lipid-lowering Treatment to Prevent Heart Attack Trial (ALLHAT) (2002) [6]	Randomized to chlorthalidone 12.5–25 mg, lisinopril 10–40 mg, amlodipine 2.5–10 mg or doxazosin 2–8 mg	42 424 patients over 55 years; BP (baseline): 146/84 mmHg; BP (chlorthalidone): 134/75 mmHg; BP (amlodipine) 135/75 mmHg; BP (lisinopril) 136/75 mmHg	Doxazosin arm discontinued due to significantly higher stroke ($P = 0.04$), heart failure ($P <0.001$) or combined CVD ($P <0.001$) compared to chlorthalidone. No differences in primary outcome for lisinopril or amlodipine compared to chlorthalidone. Higher risk of heart failure with amlodipine (RR = 1.38) or lisinopril (RR = 1.19) compared to chlorthalidone. Combined CVD (RR = 1.10) and stroke (RR = 1.15) were higher with lisinopril than chlorthalidone.

* Starting and end-titration dose range given for diuretic used.
BP = blood pressure; CHD = coronary heart disease; CV = cardiovascular; HCTZ = hydrochlorothiazide; HR = hazard ratio; MI = myocardial infarction; RR = relative risk.

CI 1–62; P = 0.05), a 64% reduction in fatal and non-fatal HF (95% CI 42–78; P <0.001) and a 34% reduction in any CV event (95% CI, 18–47; P <0.001). Blood pressure fell by 14.5±18.5 mmHg and 6.8±10.5 mmHg, in the placebo group and by 29.5±15.4 mmHg and 12.9±9.5 mmHg in the active-treatment group. While information on 24-h BP control was not reported, the fact that long-acting compounds (sustained-release indapamide and perindopril) were used would suggest that night-time BP may have been effectively reduced.

One of the most interesting diuretic-related findings was reported by investigators conducting the Multiple Risk Factor Intervention Trial (MRFIT) [22]. Patients were randomized to either Special Intervention (SI) or Usual Care (UC) with the latter receiving usual care from their physicians. The agents used as initial therapy in the SI group were either HCTZ or chlorthalidone in a dose range of 50–100 mg without specification on frequency of dosing. Of note, the choice of diuretic was not random but was made locally by the clinic staff. The initial evaluation followed 8012 men for 6.9 years and found a trend in favor of the SI group compared to the UC group but the differences were not statistically significant [22]. Six years into the trial, however, it was observed that in the nine clinics predominately using HCTZ, the mortality rate was 44% *higher* in the SI group compared to the UC group [22]. The opposite was true in the six clinics that predominately used chlorthalidone where mortality in the SI group was more favorable compared to the UC group. In response to this finding, the MRFIT Data Safety Monitoring Board changed the protocol to exclusively use chlorthalidone (daily maximum dose of 50 mg) in the SI group. In the clinics initially using HCTZ, that had a 44% *higher* mortality in the SI group, the trend reversed after the protocol change and they then had a 28% *lower* risk (P = 0.04 comparing coronary heart disease [CHD] mortality at the two time periods).

The investigators proposed several possible explanations for the fact that mortality was more favorable in the SI group at 10.5 years but not at 6.9 years of follow-up. These explanations included: a possible time delay in risk reduction that required longer follow-up in order to observe the effect or, alternatively, that the change in the protocol to switch to chlorthalidone produced the more favorable effect observed towards the end of the trial. Our recent comparative trial between HCTZ and chlorthalidone showing clear differences in 24-h BP control favoring chlorthalidone has been offered as a possible explanation for the MRFIT study findings [25, 63].

WHAT ARE THE LESSONS LEARNED FROM ALLHAT, ANBP2 AND ACCOMPLISH?

The differences between thiazide-type diuretics and other drug classes have been highlighted by the seemingly disparate findings between the ALLHAT, the Second Australian National Blood Pressure Study (ANBP2) and more recently the Avoiding Cardiovascular Events in Combination Therapy in Patients Living with Systolic Hypertension (ACCOMPLISH) trial [6, 54, 58]. The ALLHAT found significantly lower event rates for all CV disease, stroke and HF with chlorthalidone than with the ACE inhibitor lisinopril and a lower risk of heart failure with chlorthalidone than with amlodipine [6]. In contrast, the ANBP2 used HCTZ as the diuretic but found the ACE inhibitor enalapril to be superior at reducing combined morbidity and mortality, at least in men [54]. ACCOMPLISH compared the combination of HCTZ/benazepril with amlodipine/benazepril and found the CCB/ACE combination reduced CV more than the diuretic/ACE combination [58]. How could the results of these trials be so different?

The ALLHAT was a randomized, double-blind, active-controlled antihypertensive treatment trial in 42 418 patients assigned to a chlorthalidone, an ACE inhibitor (lisinopril), a CCB (amlodipine) or an α-blocker (doxazosin). The doxazosin arm was terminated early after 3.3 years of follow-up when higher rates of heart failure were observed when compared to chlorthalidone. After an average of 4.9 years of follow-up, chlorthalidone was at least as beneficial as the comparator drugs in lowering BP and preventing CV and renal outcomes and was superior for preventing HF (versus each comparator arm), combined CV events (versus α-blocker and ACE inhibitor arms), and stroke (versus ACE inhibitor [African Americans only] and α-blocker) [6].

The ANBP2 was an open-label trial in 6083 subjects treated with either diuretic-based therapy (primarily HCTZ) or an ACE inhibitor (enalapril recommended) [54]. Cardiovascular events were lower in the ACE inhibitor group (RR 0.89; 95% CI 0.79–1.00) but this difference was barely statistically significant (P = 0.05). One major difference between this study and ALLHAT was that ALLHAT had far more blacks but also eight times as many CV events as ANBP2. Because this was an open-label study with agents selected by the individual practitioners, it is not possible to determine if proper doses of HCTZ were used.

The ACCOMPLISH trial studied 11 462 high risk patients and was stopped early (42 months). Amlodipine/benazapril had a RR of 0.8 (95% CI 0.72–0.90; P = 0.0002) for major fatal and non-fatal CV events when compared to HCTZ/benazapril despite nearly identical office BPs at the end of the study. However, the composite endpoint of this study did not include HF, which is a key endpoint that has been found to be reduced by 50–68% in diuretic-based regimens [6, 20, 61]. There are other critical design features that may also explain the diuretic 'negative' findings in the ACCOMPLISH trial. First, benazepril does not have consistent 24-h BP coverage [64]. Since both regimens included benazepril, the comparison basically then is one between HCTZ and amlodipine. The study used HCTZ in suboptimal doses of only 12.5–25 mg once daily, which at best has only a 8–15 h duration of action. Amlodipine is one of the longest acting antihypertensives with a half-life of 38–50 h and provides definitive 24-h coverage [64].

Possible explanations for the differences in the findings from these three studies include differences between the populations studied, sample sizes, numbers of outcomes or the validity of outcome measures [65]. We, however, believe the differences are likely due to the inferiority of HCTZ when compared to chlorthalidone on 24-h BP control [64]. Only ALLHAT used chlorthalidone and ANBP2 and ACCOMPLISH used HCTZ in low doses given once daily. When all of the diuretic-based outcome trials are examined, those that used chlorthalidone have all been significantly different from placebo or other therapy [1, 64]. However, studies that used HCTZ have had mixed results with approximately half finding benefit and half finding either no benefit or inferior results to other drug therapy. For these reasons, we believe that chlorthalidone is the preferred thiazide diuretic. If HCTZ is used, it should be given twice daily. The only time when HCTZ once daily can be justified is within a combination regimen that clearly has 24-h BP coverage, ideally demonstrated by ambulatory BP monitoring in each specific patient.

SUMMARY

We believe that thiazide diuretics should remain preferred agents for step one therapy of hypertension in both uncomplicated hypertension and in patients with co-existing conditions. Patients with higher initial BP values or those with lower goals (e.g. diabetes, chronic kidney disease, ischemic heart disease) will likely require two or more antihypertensives. In these cases, the diuretic and the second agent should generally be started together and titrated to appropriate dosages to control BP. Future studies are necessary to determine if the differing results of ALLHAT, ANBP2 and ACCOMPLISH are due to differences in the level of 24-h BP control, especially during the night and early morning.

REFERENCES

1. Carter BL, Ernst ME, Cohen JD. Hydrochlorothiazide versus chlorthalidone: evidence supporting their interchangeability. *Hypertension* 2004; 43:4–9.
2. Cutler JA, Davis BR. Thiazide-type diuretics and beta-adrenergic blockers as first-line drug treatments for hypertension. *Circulation* 2008; 117:2691–2704; discussion 2705.
3. Messerli FH, Bangalore S, Julius S. Risk/benefit assessment of beta-blockers and diuretics precludes their use for first-line therapy in hypertension. *Circulation* 2008; 117:2706–2715; discussion 2715.
4. American Heart Association's Heart Disease and Stroke Statistics – 2008 Update. http://www.americanheart.org/statistics.
5. Chobanian AV, Bakris GL, Black HR *et al*. Seventh report of the Joint National Committee on Prevention, Detection, Evaluation, and Treatment of High Blood Pressure. *Hypertension* 2003; 42:1206–1252.
6. Major outcomes in high-risk hypertensive patients randomized to angiotensin-converting enzyme inhibitor or calcium channel blocker vs diuretic: the Antihypertensive and Lipid-Lowering Treatment to Prevent Heart Attack Trial (ALLHAT). *JAMA* 2002; 288:2981–2997.
7. Carter BL, Bergus GR, Dawson JD *et al*. A cluster randomized trial to evaluate physician/pharmacist collaboration to improve blood pressure control. *J Clin Hypertens (Greenwich)* 2008; 10:260–271.
8. Calhoun DA, Jones D, Textor S *et al*. Resistant hypertension: diagnosis, evaluation, and treatment: a scientific statement from the American Heart Association Professional Education Committee of the Council for High Blood Pressure Research. *Circulation* 2008; 117:e510–e526.
9. Davis BR, Piller LB, Cutler JA *et al*. Role of diuretics in the prevention of heart failure: the Antihypertensive and Lipid-Lowering Treatment to Prevent Heart Attack Trial. *Circulation* 2006; 113:2201–2210.
10. Einhorn PT, Davis BR, Massie BM *et al*. The Antihypertensive and Lipid Lowering Treatment to Prevent Heart Attack Trial (ALLHAT) Heart Failure Validation Study: diagnosis and prognosis. *Am Heart J* 2007; 153:42–53.
11. Psaty BM, Lumley T, Furberg CD *et al*. Health outcomes associated with various antihypertensive therapies used as first-line agents: a network meta-analysis. *JAMA* 2003; 289:2534–2544.
12. Stafford RS, Monti V, Furberg CD, Ma J. Long-term and short-term changes in antihypertensive prescribing by office-based physicians in the United States. *Hypertension* 2006; 48:213–218.
13. Ma J, Lee KV, Stafford RS. Changes in antihypertensive prescribing during US outpatient visits for uncomplicated hypertension between 1993 and 2004. *Hypertension* 2006; 48:846–852.
14. Sica DA. Diuretic-related side effects: development and treatment. *J Clin Hypertens (Greenwich)* 2004; 6:532–540.
15. Carter BL, Sica DA. Strategies to improve the cardiovascular risk profile of thiazide-type diuretics as used in the management of hypertension. *Expert Opin Drug Saf* 2007; 6:583–594.
16. The 1988 report of the Joint National Committee on Prevention, Detection, Evaluation, and Treatment of High Blood Pressure. *Arch Intern Med* 1988; 148:1023–1038.
17. The fifth report of the Joint National Committee on Prevention, Detection, Evaluation, and Treatment of High Blood Pressure (JNC V). *Arch Intern Med* 1993; 153:154–183.
18. Weber MA, Laragh JH. Hypertension: steps forward and steps backward. The Joint National Committee fifth report. *Arch Intern Med* 1993; 153:149–152.
19. The sixth report of the Joint National Committee on Prevention, Detection, Evaluation, and Treatment of High Blood Pressure. *Arch Intern Med* 1997; 157:2413–2446.
20. Beckett NS, Peters R, Fletcher AE *et al*. Treatment of hypertension in patients 80 years of age or older. *N Engl J Med* 2008; 358:1887–1898.
21. Diuretics. In: Brunton LL, Lazo JS, Parker KL, (eds). *Goodman & Gilman's The Pharmacological Basis of Therapeutics*, 11th edition. New York: McGraw-Hill Companies Inc., 2008.
22. Mortality after 10 1/2 years for hypertensive participants in the Multiple Risk Factor Intervention Trial. *Circulation* 1990; 82:1616–1628.
23. Sica DA. Chlorthalidone: has it always been the best thiazide-type diuretic? *Hypertension* 2006; 47:321–322.
24. Ernst ME, Grimm RH Jr. Thiazide diuretics: 50 years and beyond. *Curr Hypertens Rev* 2008; 4:256–265.
25. Ernst ME, Carter BL, Goerdt CJ *et al*. Comparative antihypertensive effects of hydrochlorothiazide and chlorthalidone on ambulatory and office blood pressure. *Hypertension* 2006; 47:352–358.

26. Verdecchia P, Reboldi G, Angeli F *et al.* Adverse prognostic significance of new diabetes in treated hypertensive subjects. *Hypertension* 2004; 43:963–969.

27. Carter BL, Basile J. Development of diabetes with thiazide diuretics: the potassium issue. *J Clin Hypertens (Greenwich)* 2005; 7:638–640.

28. Zillich AJ, Garg J, Basu S, Bakris GL, Carter BL. Thiazide diuretics, potassium, and the development of diabetes: a quantitative review. *Hypertension* 2006; 48:219–224.

29. Amery A, Berthaux P, Bulpitt C *et al.* Glucose intolerance during diuretic therapy. Results of trial by the European Working Party on Hypertension in the Elderly. *Lancet* 1978; 1:681–683.

30. Savage PJ, Pressel SL, Curb JD *et al.* Influence of long-term, low-dose, diuretic-based, antihypertensive therapy on glucose, lipid, uric acid, and potassium levels in older men and women with isolated systolic hypertension: The Systolic Hypertension in the Elderly Program. SHEP Cooperative Research Group. *Arch Intern Med* 1998; 158:741–751.

31. Tweeddale MG, Ogilvie RI, Ruedy J. Antihypertensive and biochemical effects of chlorthalidone. *Clin Pharmacol Ther* 1977; 22:519–527.

32. Lakshman MR, Reda DJ, Materson BJ, Cushman WC, Freis ED. Diuretics and beta-blockers do not have adverse effects at 1 year on plasma lipid and lipoprotein profiles in men with hypertension. Department of Veterans Affairs Cooperative Study Group on Antihypertensive Agents. *Arch Intern Med* 1999; 159:551–558.

33. Carter BL, Einhorn PT, Brands M *et al.* Thiazide-induced dysglycemia: call for research from a working group from the national heart, lung, and blood institute. *Hypertension* 2008; 52:30–36.

34. Barzilay JI, Davis BR, Cutler JA *et al.* Fasting glucose levels and incident diabetes mellitus in older nondiabetic adults randomized to receive 3 different classes of antihypertensive treatment: a report from the Antihypertensive and Lipid-Lowering Treatment to Prevent Heart Attack Trial (ALLHAT). *Arch Intern Med* 2006; 166:2191–2201.

35. Elliott WJ, Meyer PM. Incident diabetes in clinical trials of antihypertensive drugs: a network meta-analysis. *Lancet* 2007; 369:201–207.

36. Kostis JB, Wilson AC, Freudenberger RS, Cosgrove NM, Pressel SL, Davis BR. Long-term effect of diuretic-based therapy on fatal outcomes in subjects with isolated systolic hypertension with and without diabetes. *Am J Cardiol* 2005; 95:29–35.

37. Phillips RA. New-onset diabetes mellitus less deadly than elevated blood pressure?: following the evidence in the administration of thiazide diuretics. *Arch Intern Med* 2006; 166:2174–2176.

38. Whelton PK, Barzilay J, Cushman WC *et al.* Clinical outcomes in antihypertensive treatment of type 2 diabetes, impaired fasting glucose concentration, and normoglycemia: Antihypertensive and Lipid-Lowering Treatment to Prevent Heart Attack Trial (ALLHAT). *Arch Intern Med* 2005; 165:1401–1409.

39. Curb JD, Pressel SL, Cutler JA *et al.* Effect of diuretic-based antihypertensive treatment on cardiovascular disease risk in older diabetic patients with isolated systolic hypertension. Systolic Hypertension in the Elderly Program Cooperative Research Group. [erratum appears in JAMA 1997; 277:1356]. *JAMA* 1996; 276:1886–1892.

40. Wright JT Jr, Harris-Haywood S, Pressel S *et al.* Clinical outcomes by race in hypertensive patients with and without the metabolic syndrome: Antihypertensive and Lipid-Lowering Treatment to Prevent Heart Attack Trial (ALLHAT). *Arch Intern Med* 2008; 168:207–217.

41. Cutler JA. Thiazide-associated glucose abnormalities: prognosis, etiology, and prevention: is potassium balance the key? *Hypertension* 2006; 48:198–200.

42. Nordrehaug JE, von der Lippe G. Hypokalaemia and ventricular fibrillation in acute myocardial infarction. *Br Heart J* 1983; 50:525–529.

43. Chapman N, Dobson J, Wilson S *et al.* Effect of spironolactone on blood pressure in subjects with resistant hypertension. *Hypertension* 2007; 49:839–845.

44. Saha C, Eckert GJ, Ambrosius WT *et al.* Improvement in blood pressure with inhibition of the epithelial sodium channel in blacks with hypertension. *Hypertension* 2005; 46:481–487.

45. Weinberger MH. Influence of an angiotensin converting-enzyme inhibitor on diuretic-induced metabolic effects in hypertension. *Hypertension* 1983; 5:132–138.

46. Simunic M, Rumboldt Z, Ljutic D, Sardelic S. Ramipril decreases chlorthalidone-induced loss of magnesium and potassium in hypertensive patients. *J Clin Pharmacol* 1995; 35:1150–1155.

47. Bakris G, Molitch M, Hewkin A *et al.* Differences in glucose tolerance between fixed-dose antihypertensive drug combinations in people with metabolic syndrome. *Diabetes Care* 2006; 29:2592–2597.

48. Spiers DR, Wade RC. Double-blind parallel study of a combination of chlorthalidone 50 mg and triamterene 50 mg in patients with mild and moderate hypertension. *Curr Med Res Opin* 1996; 13:409–415.

49. Hort JF, Wilkins HM. Changes in blood pressure, serum potassium and electrolytes with a combination of triamterene and a low dose of chlorthalidone. *Curr Med Res Opin* 1991; 12:430–440.

50. Multiclinic comparison of amiloride, hydrochlorothiazide, and hydrochlorothiazide plus amiloride in essential hypertension. Multicenter Diuretic Cooperative Study Group. *Arch Intern Med* 1981; 141:482–486.

51. Myers MG. Hydrochlorothiazide with or without amiloride for hypertension in the elderly. A dose-titration study. *Arch Intern Med* 1987; 147:1026–1030.

52. Kohvakka A, Salo H, Gordin A, Eisalo A. Antihypertensive and biochemical effects of different doses of hydrochlorothiazide alone or in combination with triamterene. *Acta Med Scand* 1986; 219:381–386.

53. Larochelle P, Logan AG. Hydrochlorothiazide-amiloride versus hydrochlorothiazide alone for essential hypertension: effects on blood pressure and serum potassium level. *Can Med Assoc J* 1985; 132:801–805.

54. Wing LM, Reid CM, Ryan P *et al.* A comparison of outcomes with angiotensin-converting-enzyme inhibitors and diuretics for hypertension in the elderly. *N Engl J Med* 2003; 348:583–592.

55. Medical Research Council trial of treatment of hypertension in older adults: principal results. MRC Working Party. *BMJ* 1992; 304:405–412.

56. Leren P, Helgeland A. Oslo Hypertension Study. *Drugs* 1986; 31(suppl 1):41–45.

57. Wikstrand J, Warnold I, Olsson G, Tuomilehto J, Elmfeldt D, Berglund G. Primary prevention with metoprolol in patients with hypertension. Mortality results from the MAPHY study. *JAMA* 1988; 259:1976–1982.

58. Jamerson K, Weber MA, Bakris GL *et al.* Benazapril plus amlodipine or hydrochlorothiazide for hypertension in high-risk patients. *N Engl J Med* 2008; 359:2417–2428.

59. Five-year findings of the hypertension detection and follow-up program. I. Reduction in mortality of persons with high blood pressure, including mild hypertension. Hypertension Detection and Follow-up Program Cooperative Group. *JAMA* 1979; 242:2562–2571.

60. Five-year findings of the hypertension detection and follow-up program. III. Reduction in stroke incidence among persons with high blood pressure. Hypertension Detection and Follow-up Program Cooperative Group. *JAMA* 1982; 247:633–638.

61. Prevention of stroke by antihypertensive drug treatment in older persons with isolated systolic hypertension. Final results of the Systolic Hypertension in the Elderly Program (SHEP). SHEP Cooperative Research Group. *JAMA* 1991; 265:3255–3264.

62. Anonymous. Major cardiovascular events in hypertensive patients randomized to doxazosin vs chlorthalidone: the Antihypertensive and Lipid-Lowering Treatment to Prevent Heart Attack Trial (ALLHAT). ALLHAT Collaborative Research Group. *JAMA* 2000; 283:1967–1975.

63. Grimm R. Diuretics are preferred over angiotensin II-converting enzyme inhibitors for initial therapy of uncomplicated hypertension. *Am J Kidney Dis* 2007; 50:188–196.

64. Ernst ME, Carter BL, Basile JN. All thiazide-like diuretics are not chlorthalidone: putting the ACCOMPLISH study into perspective. *J Clin Hypertens (Greenwich)* 2009; 11:5–10.

65. Alderman MH. ALLHAT and beyond. *Am J Hypertens* 2003; 16:512–514.

66. Amery A, Birkenhager W, Brixko P *et al.* Mortality and morbidity results from the European Working Party on High Blood Pressure in the Elderly trial. *Lancet* 1985; 1:1349–1354.

67. Borhani NO, Mercuri M, Borhani PA *et al.* Final outcome results of the Multicenter Isradipine Diuretic Atherosclerosis Study (MIDAS). A randomized controlled trial. *JAMA* 1996; 276:785–791.

68. Brown MJ, Palmer CR, Castaigne A *et al.* Morbidity and mortality in patients randomised to double-blind treatment with a long-acting calcium-channel blocker or diuretic in the International Nifedipine GITS study: Intervention as a Goal in Hypertension Treatment (INSIGHT). *Lancet* 2000; 356:366–372.

69. Neaton JD, Grimm RH Jr, Prineas RJ *et al.* Treatment of Mild Hypertension Study. Final results. Treatment of Mild Hypertension Study Research Group. *JAMA* 1993; 270:713–724.

3

Are lifestyle modifications effective for the treatment of hypertension?

T. A. Kotchen, J. M. Kotchen

BACKGROUND

A poor diet and sedentary lifestyle are major contributors to hypertension, obesity, type 2 diabetes mellitus, dyslipidemia, and cardiovascular disease morbidity and mortality. Guidelines regarding diet and physical activity are key components of current recommendations for the prevention and management of hypertension. Despite the enthusiasm of professional societies and healthcare providers, some have argued that the benefits of non-pharmacologic therapy of hypertension have been overstated [1, 2]. For example, some non-pharmacologic measures may be more onerous and more expensive for a patient than taking a daily, low dose of a thiazide diuretic. Adherence to recommended lifestyle modifications may be difficult to sustain, and compliance may be difficult to assess. It has been argued that the critical approach that has been applied to evaluating the impact of drug treatment has not been applied with equal rigor to non-pharmacologic interventions. The purpose of this chapter is to address the contention that lifestyle modifications are relatively ineffective for the prevention and treatment of hypertension.

WHAT IS THE EFFECT OF OBESITY ON BLOOD PRESSURE?

Being overweight and/or obese are established risk factors for hypertension, and hypertension is approximately twice as prevalent in the obese as in the non-obese [3]. In both women and men, centrally located body fat is more closely related to blood pressure (BP) elevation than is peripheral body fat. Both general adiposity and abdominal adiposity (measured as waist circumference or waist-to-hip ratio), independent of general obesity, are associated with increased mortality [4] The association of obesity with hypertension across populations and racial/ethnic groups suggests that hypertension is causally related to obesity and that weight loss may be an effective strategy for lowering BP [5, 6].

Longitudinal studies provide compelling evidence for a causal relationship between weight gain and the subsequent development of hypertension, and a higher body mass index (BMI) at a particular age is predictive of hypertension at a later age. Recent National Health and Nutrition Examination Survey (NHANES) data indicate that the prevalence of

Theodore A. Kotchen, MD, MBA, Professor of Medicine, Medical College of Wisconsin, Milwaukee, Wisconsin, USA.

Jane Morley Kotchen, MD, MPH, Professor, Departments of Population Health and Medicine, Medical College of Wisconsin, Milwaukee, Wisconsin, USA.

both hypertension and obesity increased between 1988–1994 and 1999–2004 in the US, raising the possibility of a causal relationship [7, 8]. However, an upward shift of systolic BP was observed only in persons with a BMI <25 kg/m². Further, BP levels are correlated with various measures of adiposity in normotensive, but not in hypertensive persons [9]. These observations suggest that a potential impact of adiposity on BP is attenuated in obese, hypertensive individuals.

Short-term trials have consistently documented a reduction in BP by weight loss, independent of dietary sodium chloride (NaCl), in both hypertensive and normotensive persons. Based on pooled results of controlled dietary intervention trials, it has been estimated that a mean change in body weight of 9.2 kg is associated with a 6.3 mmHg change in systolic BP and a 3.1 mmHg change in diastolic BP [10]. Even modest weight loss (5–10% of initial weight) has a recognizable BP lowering effect. Modest weight loss, with or without NaCl reduction, can reduce the occurrence of hypertension by ~20% among overweight, pre-hypertensive individuals and can generally facilitate medication step-down and drug withdrawal [11]. Most of these trials have been relatively short term, and less information is available about the long-term effects of sustained weight loss on BP.

It is likely that predisposition of the overweight and obese individual to the development of hypertension is modulated by interactions between genes and environmental factors. Preliminary studies suggest unique genetic associations and/or linkages with obesity-related hypertension. Nevertheless, from both patient care and population perspectives, preventing obesity and encouraging weight loss for already overweight children, adolescents, and adults are prudent strategies for the prevention and treatment of hypertension.

WHAT IS THE EFFECT OF NACL INTAKE ON BLOOD PRESSURE?

A high NaCl intake convincingly contributes to elevated arterial pressure in a number of genetic and acquired models of experimental hypertension. The chimpanzee is phylogenetically close to the human and, in the chimpanzee, BPs track with relatively modest changes in dietary NaCl [12]. In humans, both observational studies and intervention trials document an association between NaCl intake and BP. In a number of populations, the prevalence of hypertension and the age-related rise of BP are related to NaCl intake [13]. As reviewed in two meta-analyses, the fall in BP with a 100 mmol fall in urinary sodium (Na⁺) (surrogate for Na⁺ intake) is more prominent in hypertensive (3.7–4.9/0.9–2.9 mmHg) than in normotensive (1.0–1.7/0.1–1.0 mmHg) persons [14, 15]. Many of the trials in these analyses were of rather short duration (<2 weeks), and the full impact of reduction in NaCl intake on BP may not have been realized. Similarly, in children and adolescents, a recent meta-analysis suggests that short-term reduction of dietary NaCl also reduces BP [16], and a cross sectional, observational study found that for each 1-gm/day intake increase of NaCl systolic BP and pulse pressure increased by 0.4 mmHg and 0.6 mmHg, respectively [17].

Although there is individual variability in BP responses to NaCl, methodologies and criteria for defining 'salt sensitivity' are arbitrary and poorly standardized. Based on results of acute NaCl depletion or acute NaCl loading protocols, 30–50% of hypertensive persons and a smaller percent of normotensive persons are estimated to be NaCl sensitive [18]. Blood pressure responsiveness to NaCl may also be modified by other components of the diet. The effect of NaCl on BP may be potentiated by diets low in calcium (Ca²⁺) or potassium (K⁺) content and attenuated by high intakes of Ca²⁺ or K⁺. Phenotypic characteristics associated with increased sensitivity to NaCl include hypertension, increased age, obesity, a history of low birth weight, and African-American race.

Animal studies provide convincing evidence of a genetic susceptibility of BP to salt sensitivity. The identification of human genetic markers of salt sensitivity is an active area of investigation. The most frequently studied genetic polymorphisms regarding salt sensitivity include: α-adducin Gly460TRP, angiotensin converting enzyme I/D, angiotensinogen M235 IT, G protein β-3 C825T, aldosterone synthase, and 11-β-hydroxysteroid dehydrogenase type 2 G534A [19]. Results among studies have been inconsistent, in part reflecting genetic heterogeneity among populations and heterogeneity in the methods for assessment of salt sensitivity.

WHAT ARE THE LONG-TERM EFFECTS OF NACL INTAKE ON CARDIOVASCULAR DISEASE?

Despite its well established relationship with cardiovascular disease, BP is but an intermediate endpoint. The most convincing case for a lifestyle modification as an effective intervention is if it both lowers BP and reduces the incidence of cardiovascular disease. Several prospective observational studies suggest that a higher NaCl intake is associated with an increased risk of subsequent cardiovascular events [20]. 'Salt sensitive' normotensive individuals may have a cumulative mortality similar to that of hypertensive patients [21]. In Finland, over a 25–30 year period, a progressive decrease in salt intake has been associated with a reduction of the BP in the population and in a 75–80% decrease in stroke and coronary heart disease mortality [22]. Based on the application of a computer-stimulation model of previously published data and the assumption that lowering BP reduces the risk of cardiovascular disease, it has been estimated that reducing dietary NaCl in the US by 3 g per day would reduce the annual incidence of coronary heart disease, stroke, myocardial infarction, and the annual number of deaths by approximately 30% [23].

Clinical trials also provide a compelling rationale for recommending avoidance of a high NaCl intake. The long-term effect of NaCl reduction on cardiovascular disease has recently been described in two large randomized trials, Trials of Hypertension Prevention) (TOHP) I and II [24]. Over 3000 participants with high normal BP (pre-hypertension) were randomized to a reduced salt group for 18 months (TOHP I) or 36–48 months (TOHP II), or to a control group. The reductions in NaCl intake were 44 mEq/day and 33 mEq/day, respectively. At 10–15 years post-trial, individuals who were originally allocated to the reduced NaCl group had a 25–30% lower incidence of cardiovascular events in both studies after adjusting for confounding factors.

WHAT OTHER DIETARY FACTORS ARE RELATED TO BLOOD PRESSURE?

Observational studies suggest a J-shaped relationship between alcohol consumption and BP [25]. Light drinkers (1–2 drinks per day) have lower BPs than teetotalers, whereas in comparison with non-drinkers, a small but significant elevation of BP is seen in persons consuming three or more drinks per day (a standard drink contains approximately 14 g of ethanol and is defined as a 12-ounce glass of beer, a 6-ounce glass of table wine, or 1.5 ounces of distilled spirits). The contribution to the prevalence of hypertension attributable to consumption of more than two drinks of alcohol per day has been estimated to be 5 to 7%. In a meta-analysis of 15 randomized controlled trials, reduction of alcohol intake was associated with significant reductions of mean (95% confidence interval) systolic and diastolic BPs of –3.31 mmHg (–2.52 to –4.10 mmHg) and –2.04 mmHg (–1.49 to –2.58 mmHg), respectively. A dose–response relationship was observed between mean percent alcohol reduction and mean BP reduction. Blood pressure reductions were greater in those with higher baseline BPs [26].

Results of observational studies suggest an inverse relationship between BP and dietary intakes of K^+, Ca^{2+}, and magnesium (Mg^{2+}) [11, 27]. Populations that consume lower amounts of these minerals tend to have higher BP levels and a higher prevalence of hypertension. However, in controlled clinical trials, provision of these minerals as supplements has had little or no consistent effect on BP. Consequently, there is no justification for recommending K^+, Ca^{2+}, or Mg^{2+} supplements for the prevention or treatment of hypertension. Nevertheless, adequate amounts of these substances should be included in the diet for overall health. For example, higher Ca^{2+} intakes are recommended for osteoporosis prevention, and lower K^+ intakes are associated with an increased incidence of stroke deaths [28]. Although fruits and vegetables are the best sources of K^+, (as opposed to dietary supplements of K^+) it remains to be determined whether the BP-lowering capacity of fruits, vegetables, and low fat dairy products can be explained entirely by their electrolyte content.

WHAT ARE THE EFFECTS OF OVERALL DIET ON BLOOD PRESSURE AND CARDIOVASCULAR DISEASE?

From a pragmatic perspective, recommendations about nutrition for the prevention and treatment of hypertension should address overall diet rather than any single nutrient. Results of both observational studies and intervention trials demonstrate that lacto-ovo vegetarian diets are associated with lower BP levels and a decreased incidence of hypertension than is the case with omnivorous diets. Further, several prospective observational studies suggest that consumption of diets high in fruit and vegetable content are associated with a lesser BP increase with aging [29]. The specific nutrients responsible for the BP reduction associated with vegetarian diets have not been defined.

The Dietary Approaches to Stop Hypertension (DASH) trial was a randomized multi-center study that evaluated the effects of three dietary patterns over 8 weeks on BP in 459 adults with high normal BP or mild hypertension [30]. The dietary interventions were as follows:

(a) Control diet
(b) A diet rich in fruits and vegetables
(c) A "combination" diet rich in fruits and vegetables and low fat dairy products

NaCl content was 8 g/day in all three diets. Systolic and diastolic BPs were significantly reduced with the fruit and vegetable diet (-2.5 and -1 mmHg, respectively) compared with the control diet; blood pressures were reduced to a greater extent by the combination diet (-5.5 and -3.0 mmHg, respectively). The BP lowering effect of the DASH diet was more pronounced in hypertensives than in non-hypertensives and greater in black than in white participants. In a subsequent study, three levels of Na^+ intake (50, 100, 150 mEq/day) were evaluated for 30 days each in 412 persons consuming either the combination-DASH diet or a control diet [31]. A significant BP decrease occurred on the lower Na^+ intakes in participants following either the DASH or control diet. The combined effects of the DASH low-Na^+ diet lowered systolic and diastolic BP by 8.9 and 4.5 mmHg, respectively, compared with the high-Na^+ phase of the control diet. DASH-like diets have also been shown to reduce BP in adults with pre-hypertension or Stage 1 hypertension [11, 32, 33] and in adolescents with elevated BP [34].

In several recent observational studies and clinical trials, the outcomes with healthy eating patterns have been mixed. In a national US cohort of individuals aged 45 years and older, dietary patterns similar to the DASH diet were associated with decreased mortality [35]. The Nurses Health Study demonstrated a decreased risk of cardiovascular disease and stroke in middle-aged women who consumed a DASH-like diet [36], whereas the Iowa Women's Health Study failed to demonstrate an independent association between the consumption of a DASH-like diet and reduced risk for hypertension or cardiovascular disease mortality [37]. In the Women's Health Initiative, over a mean of 8.1 years of follow-up, a dietary intervention that reduced fat intake and increased fruits, vegetables, and grains did not significantly reduce the risk of coronary heart disease, stroke, or cardiovascular disease in post-menopausal women [38]. In the Women's Health Initiative trial, there was no significant reduction of systolic BP and only a small reduction of diastolic BP (<1 mmHg).

Limited clinical trial data are available concerning the combined effect of diet, weight loss, and exercise on BP. The Diet, Exercise and Weight-loss Intervention Trial (DEW-IT) randomized 44 overweight adults to a lifestyle group or control group [39]. For 9 weeks the lifestyle group received a hypocaloric version of the DASH diet, containing 100 mEq/day of Na$^+$. This group also participated in a moderate-intensity exercise program three times per week. The lifestyle group experienced significantly greater reductions in weight (4.9 kg) and mean 24-hour BPs (9.5/5.3 mmHg) compared with the control group.

WHAT IS THE ROLE OF PHYSICAL ACTIVITY IN HYPERTENSION PREVENTION AND CONTROL?

Physical activity is a useful adjunct for the prevention and treatment of hypertension. In a classical study of almost 15 000 Harvard male graduates, alumni who did not engage in vigorous sports play were at 35% greater risk of developing hypertension than those who did [40]. Lack of physical activity predicted an increased risk of hypertension. Other large observational studies have also described an inverse relationship between BP and either habitual physical activity or measured physical fitness. Physically active individuals live longer. In a meta-analysis of 54 randomized controlled trials, which included 2419 subjects, regular aerobic exercise was associated with an overall, pooled reduction in BP of 3.8/2.6 mmHg [41]. Similar BP reductions were observed in normotensive and hypertensive persons, and the association between exercise and BP reduction was independent of weight change. Trials with longer follow-up (>24 weeks) had a smaller effect than trials of shorter duration, possibly due to decreased participant adherence to the exercise regimen in the longer trials. At least 120 minutes per week of aerobic activity of moderate intensity (e.g. brisk walking) appears to be needed for a clinically relevant BP effect.

WHAT IS THE ROLE OF RELAXATION TRAINING IN HYPERTENSION CONTROL?

Several recent reviews have indicated that psychosocial stress is an independent risk factor for both hypertension and myocardial infarction. Consequently, there is increasing interest in the potential value of relaxation techniques for hypertension prevention and treatment. Recent meta-analyses, however, have shown that simple biofeedback, relaxation-assisted biofeedback, progressive muscle relaxation, and stress management training do not significantly and consistently reduce elevated BP. In contrast, in clinical trials led by investigators at the Maharishi Institute of Natural Medicine and Prevention, Transcendental Meditation (TM) resulted in BP reductions of 5.0/2.8 mmHg in hypertensive persons [42]. Transcendental meditation is described as *"a unique and effortless process of taking the attention to successively finer states of a thought, until thought is transcended and the mind experiences pure awareness."* Instruction in TM requires a qualified teacher who is certified through the Maharishi Vedic Education Foundation. Additionally, pooled data (202 patients) from two randomized, controlled trials that included the TM program as well as other behavioral stress-decreasing interventions found that in subjects with elevated BP (average follow-up of 7.6 years) a 23% lower all-cause mortality rate and a 30% lower cardiovascular disease mortality rate in the TM group than in controls [43].

WHAT ARE THE MOST EFFECTIVE STRATEGIES FOR SUCCESSFUL INCORPORATION OF RECOMMENDED LIFESTYLE INTERVENTIONS FOR THE PREVENTION AND TREATMENT OF HYPERTENSION?

A large number of behavioral intervention trials have tested the effects of weight loss and dietary change on BP. The interventions in many of these trials were based on social cognitive theory, self-applied behavior modification techniques, the relapse prevention model, and the transtheoretical or stages-of-change model [11]. Characteristic findings are successful behavior change over the short term, typically 6 months, with subsequent recidivism. For example, approximately two-thirds of persons who lose weight will regain it within one year, and almost all persons who lose weight will regain it within five years [44]. Dietary counseling and lifestyle modifications are the primary approaches for treating and preventing obesity, and their impact is relatively modest. A recent meta-analysis of randomized, controlled trials found that dietary-counseling-based weight loss programs produced a mean net treatment effect of approximately two body mass index units (6% of initial body weight) of weight loss at 1 year compared with usual care interventions [45]. The treatment effect of the intervention tended to diminish over time. Continued personal contact interactions seem to be more effective than self-monitoring of dietary intake or than interactions based on interactive technology [46].

Increased physical activity is a useful adjunct in the treatment of obesity, and physical activity or planned exercise should be an important component of any weight loss plan to prevent hypertension or reduce BP. For example, incorporation of 30 minutes of aerobic exercise into daily activities should be a long-term goal. Behavioral intervention studies suggest that initial changes in activity levels of sedentary people should employ simple, moderate-intensity activities such as brisk walking. Physical activity also increases the general sense of well-being.

Depending on the degree of obesity, the refractoriness to non-pharmacologic therapy, and the associated comorbidities and cardiovascular risk factors, pharmacologic therapy or bariatric surgery may be recommended. Sibutramine (a serotonin and noradrenalaine reuptake inhibitor) and orlistat (a gastrointestinal lipase inhibitor) are able to produce a mean weight loss of 10% of initial weight. In contrast to orlistat, sibutramine may be associated with small increases of BP although sometimes with BP reduction if weight loss is significant enough.

Adherence to recommended reductions of NaCl intake is generally low. Simple advice provided at healthcare settings has low effectiveness. With intensive counseling, only 20–40% of participants in relatively short term Na^+ reduction trials reduce their Na^+ intake to below the recommended upper limit of 2400 mg/day [47]. In the DASH study, diets with low or intermediate NaCl content were acceptable to adults with pre-hypertension and stage 1 hypertension. However, this was a short-term trial (30 days on each of three NaCl intakes) and all food was provided to study participants. In short-term trials, group and individual counseling sessions have also been effective in improving adherence to a DASH dietary regimen in adults and adolescents with pre-hypertension or stage 1 hypertension [33]. Intervention strategies included clinic and telephone/mail-based behavioral interventions.

The limited long-term success of intensive behavioral intervention programs highlights the importance of environmental changes to facilitate adoption of recommended lifestyle interventions. Potential barriers to the adoption of healthier diets include expense and the fact that >75% of consumed salt is hidden in processed foods. A meaningful strategy to reduce NaCl intake should involve cooperation of food manufacturers and restaurants. For example, in the United Kingdom, the Food Standards Agency (FSA) is working with the food industry to voluntarily and gradually lower the salt content of processed foods. Progress to date has been encouraging. A similar strategy might be adopted in the US.

WHY NOT RECOMMEND ANTIHYPERTENSIVE DRUG THERAPY AS AN ALTERNATIVE TO LIFESTYLE MODIFICATIONS?

Some observers have questioned the advantage of lifestyle interventions, rather than drug therapy, to lower BP [1, 2]. To answer this question, it is appropriate to separately consider hypertensive individuals and the general population. Among hypertensive patients, although lifestyle modifications alone, in the absence of drug therapy, may not be sufficient to lower BP to recommended target levels, this is not a rationale for ignoring the contribution of healthy lifestyles to overall morbidity and mortality. Hypertension is frequently associated with additional cardiovascular disease risk factors, and clustering of risk factors increases the likelihood of subsequent morbidity and mortality [48]. The constellation of hypertension, dyslipidemia, centripetal obesity, and insulin resistance with impaired glucose metabolism

Table 3.1 Lifestyle recommendations for the prevention and treatment of hypertension (adapted with permission from [11, 50, 51]).

- Maintain body weight in a healthy range (BMI 18.5–24.9 kg/m^2); prevent gradual weight gain over time.
- Consume <2400 mg sodium per day (<6 g NaCl); consume <1500 mg sodium per day if hypertensive, black, middle-aged or older (strategies include: read food labels; avoid use of table salt; reduce salt used in food preparation; use herbs and spices for flavoring meats and vegetables instead of salt; limit intake of processed foods; avoid salty foods such as processed meat and fish, pickles, soy sauce, salted nuts, chips and other snack foods).
- Consume a diet rich in fruits, vegetables, and low fat dairy products with a reduced content of saturated and total fat.
- Limit alcohol consumption (no more than two drinks per day in men and no more than one drink per day in women).
- Engage in regular aerobic physical activity (e.g. brisk walking for at least 30 minutes per day).

constitute the metabolic syndrome, and this constellation of findings occurs in approximately 50% of hypertensive patients. Lifestyle interventions should address overall cardiovascular disease risk, not simply elevated BP. These interventions are important adjuncts to the pharmacologic treatment of hypertension. Furthermore, with the adoption of recommended lifestyles, lower doses of fewer antihypertensive agents may be required to achieve BP goals, thus reducing drug-related costs and risk of medication-related side-effects. For non-hypertensive individuals, NaCl restriction and/or weight loss may be important strategies for hypertension prevention. Results of the INTERSALT study indicate that lower NaCl intake attenuates the age-related increase of BP; for populations, a 100 mEq/day lower sodium intake is associated with attenuation of the rise in systolic BP by 10 mmHg in persons aged 25–55 years [13].

Epidemiologic data support a continuous, incremental risk of cardiovascular disease, stroke, and renal disease across levels of both systolic and diastolic BP, extending down to systolic BPs below 120 mmHg [49]. Consequently, at the population level (including individuals not considered candidates for antihypertensive drug therapy), it has been projected that even an apparently small reduction of BP could have a considerable beneficial impact. For example, it has been estimated that a 3 mmHg reduction of systolic BP could lead to an 8% reduction in stroke mortality and a 5% reduction in mortality from coronary heart disease [11].

Finally, modeling healthy lifestyles may have a positive impact on other residents of a community, whereas without appropriate role models unhealthy life styles may be the norm. For example, the Center for Disease Control (CDC) has recently reported that Huntington, West Virginia is the *"unhealthiest city in America"* [50]. Huntington is a blue collar, predominantly Caucasian community with a high poverty rate. Nearly half of the adults in the five-county metropolitan area are obese, and Huntington leads the country in heart disease and diabetes mellitus. Of all US metropolitan and micropolitan statistical areas, Huntington also has the highest prevalence of persons who were told by a health professional that their BP is high (38.1%, reported in CDC 2003 Behavioral Risk Factor Surveillance System). Compared to the rest of the country, a high proportion of Huntington's population does not exercise, and the rate of smoking is high. News reports of interviews with area residents describe prevailing apathy about improving health. These statistics clearly document the unfortunate consequences, at the population level, of the failure to adopt healthy lifestyles.

SUMMARY

Evidence is overwhelming that the adoption of healthy lifestyles (summarized in Table 3.1) considerably reduces the burden of hypertension and cardiovascular disease [51, 52].

Unfortunately, adherence to these recommendations is low among the US population. For the primary prevention of cardiovascular disease, it is important that healthy lifestyles be established at a young age. Effective strategies will require a multifaceted approach for dealing with the population as a whole, targeted subgroups, and individuals with cardiovascular disease risk factors and/or clinically evident cardiovascular disease. Strategies that are based on an understanding of the process of behavioral change should assist in motivating people to make enduring lifestyle changes. In the future, genetic studies may identify those individuals who are most likely to benefit from a specific lifestyle intervention. However, enthusiasm for the adoption of healthy lifestyles should not preclude antihypertensive drug therapy. For the majority of patients with hypertension, healthy lifestyles should be regarded as useful adjuncts, not alternatives, to drug therapy.

REFERENCES

1. Nicholson DJ, Diskinson HO, Campbell F *et al*. Lifestyle interventions or drugs for patients with essential hypertension: a systematic review. *J Hypertens* 2004; 22:2043–2048.
2. Ebrahim S, Smith GD. Lowering blood pressure: a systematic review of sustained effects of non-pharmacological interventions. *J Public Health Med* 1998; 20:441–448.
3. Mertens IL, Van Gaal LF. Overweight, obesity, and blood pressure: the effects of modest weight reduction. *Obes Res* 2000; 8:270–278.
4. Pischon T, Boeing H, Hoffmann K *et al*. General and abdominal adiposity and risk of death in Europe. *N Engl J Med* 2008; 359:2105–2120.
5. Neter JE, Stam BE, Kok FJ *et al*. Influence of weight reduction on blood pressure: a meta-analysis of randomized controlled trials. *Hypertension* 2003; 52:878–884.
6. Harsha DW, Bray GA. Weight loss and blood pressure control (Pro). *Hypertension* 2008; 51:1426–1434.
7. Hajjar IM, Kotchen TA. Trends in prevalence, awareness, treatment, and control of hypertension in the United States, 1988–2000. *JAMA* 2003; 290:199–206.
8. Cutler JA, Sorlie PD, Wolz M *et al*. Trends in hypertension prevalence, awareness, treatment, and control rates in United States adults between 1988–1994 and 1999–2000. *Hypertension* 2008; 52:818–827.
9. Kotchen TA, Grim CE, Kotchen JM *et al*. Altered relationship of blood pressure to adiposity in hypertension. *Am J Hypertens* 2008; 21:284–289.
10. MacMahon SW, Cutler J, Brittan E *et al*. Obesity and hypertension: epidemiological and clinical issues. *Eur Heart J* 1987; 8(suppl B):57–70.
11. Appel LJ, Brands MW, Daniels SR *et al*. Dietary approaches to prevent and treat hypertension: a scientific statement from the American Heart Association. *Hypertension* 2006; 47:296–308.
12. Elliott P, Walker LL, Little MP *et al*. Change of salt intake affects blood pressure of chimpanzees: implications for human populations. *Circulation* 2007; 116:1563–1568.
13. Elliott P, Stamler J, Nichols R *et al*. Intersalt revisited: further analyses of 24 hour sodium excretion and blood pressure within and across populations. Intersalt Cooperative Research Group. *BMJ* 1996; 312:1249–1253.
14. Cutler JA, Follmann D, Elliott P *et al*. An overview of randomized trials of sodium reduction and blood pressure. *Hypertension* 1991; 17(suppl I):27–33.
15. Midgley JP, Matthew AG, Greenwood CM *et al*. Effect of reduced dietary sodium on blood pressure: a meta-analysis of randomized controlled trials. *JAMA* 1996; 275:1590–1597.
16. He FJ, MacGregor GA. Importance of salt in determining blood pressure in children: meta-analysis of controlled trials. *Hypertension* 2006; 48:861–869.
17. He FJ, Marrero NM, MacGregor GA. Salt and blood pressure in children and adolescents. *J Hum Hypertens* 2008; 22:4–11.
18. Weinberger MH, Miller JH, Luft FC *et al*. Definitions and characteristics of sodium sensitivity and blood pressure resistance. *Hypertension* 1986; 8(suppl II):127–134.
19. Beeks E, Dessels AGH, Kroon AA, van der Klauw MM, de Leeuw PW. Genetic predisposition to salt-sensitivity: a systematic review. *J Hypertens* 2004; 22:1243–1249.
20. Cappucio FP. Salt and cardiovascular disease. *BMJ* 2007; 334:859–860.
21. Weinberger MH, Fineberg NS, Fineberg SE *et al*. Salt sensitivity, pulse pressure, and death in normal and hypertensive humans. *Hypertension* 2001; 37:429–432.

22. Karppanen H, Mervaala E. Sodium intake and hypertension. *Prog Cardiovasc Dis* 2006; 49:59–75.
23. Bibbins-Domingo K, Chertow GM, Coxson PG *et al.* Projected effect of dietary salt reductions on future cardiovascular disease. *N Engl J Med* 2010; (10.1056/NEJMoa0907355).
24. Cook NR, Cutler JA, Obarzanek E *et al.* Long term effects of dietary sodium reduction on cardiovascular disease outcomes: observational follow-up on the trials of hypertension prevention (TOHP). *BMJ* 2007; 334:885–892.
25. Sesso HD, Cook NR, Buring JE *et al.* Alcohol consumption and the risk of hypertension in women and men. *Hypertension* 2008; 51:1080–1087.
26. Xin X, He J, Frontini MG *et al.* Effects of alcohol reduction on blood pressure: a meta-analysis of randomized controlled trials. *Hypertension* 2001; 38:1112–1117.
27. Kotchen TA, McCarron DA. Dietary electrolytes and blood pressure: a statement for healthcare professionals from the American Heart Association Nutrition Committee. *Circulation* 1998; 98:613–617.
28. Khaw KT, Barrett-Connor E. Dietary potassium and stroke-associated mortality. A 12-year prospective population study. *New Engl J Med* 1987; 316:235–240.
29. Dauchet L, Kesse-Guyot E, Czernichow S *et al.* Dietary patterns and blood pressure change over 5-y follow-up in the SU.VI.MAX cohort. *Am J Clin Nutr* 2007; 85:1650–1656.
30. Appel LJ, Moore TJ, Obarzanek E *et al.* A clinical trial of the effects of dietary patterns on blood pressure. *N Engl J Med* 1997; 336:1117–1124.
31. Sacks FM, Svetkey LP, Vollmer WM *et al.* Effects on blood pressure of reduced dietary sodium and the dietary approaches to stop hypertension (DASH) diet. *N Engl J Med* 2001; 344:3–10.
32. Appel LJ, Champagne CM, Harsha DW *et al.* Effects of comprehensive lifestyle modification on blood pressure control: main results of the PREMIER clinical trial. *JAMA* 2003; 289:2083–2093.
33. Elmer PJ, Obarzanek E, Vollmer WM *et al.* Effects of comprehensive lifestyle modification on diet, weight, physical fitness, and blood pressure control: 18-month results of a randomized trial. *Ann Int Med* 2006; 144:485–495.
34. Couch SC, Saelens BE, Levin L *et al.* The efficacy of a clinic-based behavioral nutrition intervention emphasizing a DASH-type diet for adolescents with elevated blood pressure. *J Pediatr* 2008; 154:494–501.
35. Kant AK, Graubard BI, Schatzkin A. Dietary patterns predict mortality in a national cohort: the National Health Interview Surveys, 1987 and 1992. *J Nutr* 2004; 134:1793–1799.
36. Fung TT, Chiuve SE, McCullough Ml *et al.* Adherence to a DASH-style diet and risk of coronary heart disease and stroke in women. *Arch Intern Med* 2008; 168:713–720.
37. Folsom AR, Parker ED, Harnack LJ. Degree of concordance with DASH diet guidelines and incidence of hypertension and fatal cardiovascular disease. *Am J Hypertens* 2007; 20:225–232.
38. Howard BV, Van Horn L, Hsia J *et al.* Low-fat dietary pattern and risk of cardiovascular disease. The Women's Health Initiative Randomized Controlled Dietary Modification Trial. *JAMA* 2006; 295:655–666.
39. Miller ER III, Erlinger TP, Young DR *et al.* Results of the diet, exercise, and weight loss intervention trial (DEW-IT). *Hypertension* 2002; 40:612–618.
40. Paffenbarger RS, Wing AL, Hyde RT *et al.* Physical activity and incidence of hypertension in college alumni. *Am J Epidemiol* 1983; 117:245–257.
41. Whelton SP, Chin A, Xin X *et al.* Effect of aerobic exercise on blood pressure: a meta-analysis of randomized controlled trials. *Ann Intern Med* 2002; 136:493–503.
42. Rainforth MV, Schneider RH, Nidich SI *et al.* Stress reduction programs in patients with elevated blood pressure: a systemic review and meta-analysis. *Curr Hypertens Rep* 2007; 9:520–528.
43. Schneider RH, Alexander CN, Staggers F *et al.* Long-term effects of stress reduction on mortality in person > 55 years of age with systemic hypertension. *Am J Cardiol* 2005; 95:1060–1064.
44. Methods for voluntary weight loss and control: NIH Technology Assessment Conference Panel: Consensus Development Conference, 30 March to 1 April 1992. *Ann Intern Med* 1993; 119:764–770.
45. Dansinger ML, Tatsioni A, Wong JB. Meta-analysis: the effect of dietary counseling for weight loss. *Ann Intern Med* 2007; 147:41–50.
46. Svetkey LP, Steven VJ, Brantley PJ *et al.* Comparison of strategies for sustaining weight loss: the weight loss maintenance randomized controlled trial. *JAMA* 2008; 299:1139–1148.
47. Karanja N, Lancaster KJ, Vollmer WM *et al.* Acceptability of sodium-reduced research diets, including the dietary approaches to stop hypertension diet, among adults with prehypertension and stage 1 hypertension. *J Am Diet Assoc* 2007; 107:1530–1538.

48. McNeill AM, Rosamond WD, Girman CJ *et al*. The metabolic syndrome and 11-year risk of incident cardiovascular disease in the Atherosclerosis Risk in Communities Study. *Diabetes Care* 2005; 28:385–390.

49. Kannel WB, Vasan RS, Levy D. Is the relation of systolic blood pressure to risk of cardiovascular disease continuous and graded or are there critical values? *Hypertension* 2003; 42:453–456.

50. Stobbe M. Heavy and unhealthy: nation's most obese city shrugs off distinction. *Milw J Sentinel* 2008: 1.

51. The Seventh Report of the Joint National Committee on Prevention, Detection, Evaluation, and Treatment of High Blood Pressure. *JAMA* 2003; 289:2560–2572.

52. 2005 US Dietary Guidelines. http://www.health.gov/dietaryguidelines/dgc2005/document/html.

4

Identification and management of hypertensive nephropathy

B. Burney, G. L. Bakris

BACKGROUND

Chronic kidney disease (CKD) is a major public-health problem [1] and affects approximately 14.8% of the US population [2]. It is defined as kidney damage present for at least 3 months with confirmation by biopsy or an estimated glomerular filtration rate (eGFR) <60 mL/min or the presence of albuminuria [3]. Hypertension is a well-recognized cause of CKD and 80–85% of patients with CKD have hypertension [4]. Hypertension accelerates progression of CKD and increases the associated cardiovascular morbidity and mortality [5]. Aggressive management of blood pressure (BP) focused on achieving guideline goals is critical to the slowing of CKD progression as well as to reduce the morbidity and mortality secondary to cerebrovascular and cardiovascular disease [6, 7].

The recent increase in the incidence and prevalence of hypertension correlates with the increase in prevalence of CKD. Hypertension is also the second most common cause of end-stage renal disease (ESRD) rivaled only by diabetes mellitus (DM) [2]. The presence of early stage CKD is also one of the more common medical causes for refractory or difficult to treat hypertension [8, 9].

ALBUMINURIA AS A TARGET OF NEPHROPATHY

The appearance of low levels of albuminuria, (i.e. microalbuminuria) originally thought to be the earliest sign of nephropathy (termed incipient nephropathy), is also a marker of cardiovascular risk [3, 10]. Microalbuminuria is defined as urine albumin excretion of 30–300 mg/day in a 24-h urine collection or 30–300 mg/g creatinine on a spot urine sample. Unlike microalbuminuria, macroalbuminuria, defined as >200 mg/day of albumin or >300 mg/day of protein, is indicative of overt nephropathy [10, 11].

Current guidelines from the National Kidney Foundation [3], the 2007 European Society of Hypertension (ESH)/European Society of Cardiology (ESC) [12] and the JNC-7 recommend annual screening for microalbuminuria in all groups at high cardiovascular risk, such as those with DM or kidney disease [13].

Evidence for microalbuminuria as a marker of cardiovascular risk comes from several *post hoc* analyses of trials and is further supported by meta-analyses. The Heart Outcomes

Basil Burney, MD, Fellow in Hypertension, University of Chicago, Pritzker School of Medicine, Chicago, Illinois, USA.

George L. Bakris, MD, HonD, FASN, FAHA, Professor of Medicine, Director, Hypertensive Diseases Unit, University of Chicago, Pritzker School of Medicine, Chicago, Illinois, USA.

Prevention Evaluation (HOPE) trial found that any degree of albuminuria is a risk factor for cardiovascular events in individuals with or without DM. Thus, patients with other risk factors for cardiovascular disease (e.g. hyperlipidemia and the metabolic syndrome, smoking, obesity) should routinely be screened for microalbuminuria [14]. Additionally, meta-analyses have shown microalbuminuria to be more predictive than high sensitivity C-reactive protein (hs-CRP) for cardiovascular events [11, 15].

The question as to whether albuminuria reduction should also be a target for level of BP reduction is currently debated. There are no trials in patients with CKD and microalbuminuria that specifically show a benefit of lowering the level of albuminuria, beyond that achieved with BP reduction. A recent meta-analysis firmly supports this assertion as do a number of *post hoc* analyses of individual trials [16–18].

Conversely, patients with >300 mg of albuminuria daily uniformly demonstrate slower nephropathy progression when BP is reduced below 130/80 mmHg with antihypertensive regimens including blockers of the renin-angiotensin system (RAS). A review of *post hoc* analyses of all nephropathy studies supports the notion that a greater than 30% reduction in baseline albuminuria at six months is associated with a slower decline in kidney function relative to that assumed to occur with BP reduction [11]. A *post hoc* analysis of the Reduction of Endpoints in NIDDM with the Angiotensin II Antagonist Losartan (RENAAL) study demonstrated that ESRD risk was dependent on the residual level of albuminuria, even in patients who reached the systolic BP target. This study encapsulates what others have shown, i.e. in people with advanced proteinuric kidney disease, both BP and albuminuria must be reduced to optimally reduce the risk of decline in kidney function [19]. A number of studies support this association regardless of whether the kidney disease is associated with DM as an etiology [20, 21]. This should send a message to clinicians that whenever a patient with hypertension is seen, not only should BP be a target, but albuminuria should also be assessed with spot morning urine for albumin:creatinine to then be a target for therapy. An albuminuria level above 200 mg/g creatinine should alert the clinician that BP reducing strategies should be aimed at both BP and albuminuria reduction. A recheck of albuminuria every six months as per guideline recommendations is indicated in those with advanced nephropathy [3].

GOAL BLOOD PRESSURE IN CKD

The current JNC-7 and ESH/ESC guidelines recommend a BP goal of <130/80 mmHg for patients with DM or CKD [12, 13]. The evidence to support this goal, however, is entirely based on retrospective analyses of clinical trials, with no positive prospective data available as of this writing.

In patients with DM, the current BP goal has been established mainly by results of two outcome trials that assigned patients to different goal BP levels, the United Kingdom Prospective Diabetes Study (UKPDS) and the Hypertension Optimal Treatment (HOT) trial [22, 23]. The UKPDS showed reduced cardiovascular mortality among those randomized to the lower BP goal (less than 150/85 mmHg), but the achieved BP in this group was but 144/82 mmHg, hardly the currently recommended <130/80 mmHg for patients with hypertension and diabetes. In the HOT trial, the main trial showed no benefit of lower BP in the primary analysis but a secondary analysis in the subgroup with DM (1501/18 790 patients) showed fewer cardiovascular events in those randomized to a goal diastolic BP <80 mmHg. In HOT, however, the lower BP treatment group averaged a pressure of 136/81 mmHg, not <130/80 mmHg. The results of these trials coupled with other retrospective analyses are the basis for the recommended BP goal of <130/80 mmHg. However, the trial that will definitively answer this question, the Action to Control Cardiovascular Risk in Diabetes (ACCORD trial), is as yet unfinished [24]. It is unclear if a BP goal <130/80 mmHg is optimal for retarding progression of CKD or reducing cardiovascular risk. The available data overwhelmingly supports a goal of <140/90 mmHg but not the currently recommended goal [7].

The Modification of Diet in Renal Disease (MDRD) study was the first trial that examined whether low BP goals in non-diabetic, CKD patients slowed nephropathy progression. In this study patients were assigned to a low BP group (mean arterial pressure (MAP) <92 mmHg if older than age 60 years and 98 mmHg or less for age >60 years) and a usual BP group (MAP 107 mmHg or less for age <60 years and 113 mmHg for age >60 years). At the end of the study those with a baseline level of proteinuria >1000 mg/day in the low BP group had a significant reduction in proteinuria and slowing of nephropathy when compared to the patients assigned to the usual BP group [25]. Unfortunately, this subgroup was the only one with positive results at study's end [26]. However, Sarnak and colleagues performed a *post hoc* analysis of data obtained 7 years after the end of the MDRD trial and demonstrated that the composite outcome of kidney failure and all-cause mortality were significantly lower in the lower BP group when compared to the usual BP group [27].

The only other prospective trial to examine the level of BP control on kidney disease progression was the African-American Study of Kidney Disease and Hypertension (AASK). In this trial African-American patients with hypertensive kidney disease were randomized to either a low BP goal (MAP <92 mmHg) or usual BP levels (MAP between 102 and 107 mmHg). The results of this trial demonstrated no additional benefit of achieving a lower BP goal for reducing decline in kidney disease progression when compared to the usual BP goal [28]. Moreover, upon an additional five years of follow-up on ACE inhibition and with BP levels averaging 129/78 mmHg these patients showed a slowing but not halting of nephropathy progression [29]. Like all other studies to date, AASK did show in a *post hoc* analysis therapy-related slowing of kidney disease progression in a small subset of patients who had proteinuria more than 1000 mg/day [20].

These clinical trial data are further supported by a meta-analysis of studies in non-diabetic kidney disease by the ACE Inhibition in Progressive Renal Disease (AIPRI) Study Group, which showed that the patients with systolic BP values in the 110–129 mmHg range were associated with the lowest risk of kidney disease progression in patients with urinary protein excretion >1 g/day [30].

Taken together, the current evidence fail to support a compelling argument to lower BP to <130/80 mmHg, except for those with advanced proteinuric nephropathy regardless of etiology. Hence, until the ACCORD results are available, the current evidence from appropriately powered prospective studies supports the notion that we should strive for a BP goal of <140/90 mmHg in all patients with either DM and/or kidney disease. Strong consideration, however, should be given to lowering BP to below 130/80 mmHg in patients with >1 gram of proteinuria until specific randomized trials are undertaken to clarify this issue.

IDENTIFICATION AND TREATMENT OF HYPERTENSIVE NEPHROPATHY

There are no specific symptoms associated with hypertensive nephropathy; the diagnosis is based on history, physical examination, and biochemical findings. A long-term history of poorly controlled hypertension along with an estimated glomerular filtration rate (eGFR) of <60 ml/min in the absence of >2 grams of proteinuria and DM is perhaps the most compelling evidence for hypertensive nephropathy [31].

APPROACHES TO TREATMENT

NON-PHARMACOLOGIC MEASURES

Non-pharmacologic measures play an important role in the management of hypertensive nephropathy by both reducing proteinuria and lowering BP. Lifestyle changes such as weight loss, decreasing sodium intake, exercise, smoking cessation and moderating alcohol intake are important primary or adjunctive measures that result in a reduction in BP (Table 4.1).

Table 4.1 Lifestyle modification proven to reduce blood pressure recommended by the JNC-7.

Modification	*Approximate SBP reduction (range)*
Weight reduction	5–20 mmHg/10 kg weight loss
Adopt DASH eating plan	8–14 mmHg
Dietary sodium reduction	2–8 mmHg
Physical activity	4–9 mmHg
Moderation of alcohol consumption	2–4 mmHg
SBP = systolic blood pressure.	

Salt restriction is one of the most important components of the lifestyle modifications important to BP reduction in the patient with CKD [12]. Patients with CKD are more prone to develop high BP in response to a salt load when compared to patients with normal renal function. This is due to an increase in extracellular volume after a salt load and inability of the impaired kidney to deal with this volume expansion. High salt diets (i.e. >7 g/day) also increase the oncotic pressure of the glomerular filtrate, which further exacerbates proteinuria. Furthermore, high sodium intake attenuates the effects of anti hypertensive medications while a low dietary sodium intake (2–4 g/day) helps reduce proteinuria and BP. Other than for exercise, sodium restriction has perhaps the most robust database to support its widespread adoption in clinical practice.

PHARMACOLOGIC THERAPY

The pharmacologic approach to treating hypertensive nephropathy should be to focus on achieving goal BP and NOT on the specific **class of agent** used. Clearly, there are classes of antihypertensive agents that are better tolerated than others and, hence, may improve patient adherence, but in normoalbuminuric or microalbuminuric kidney disease, there are no agents found to be superior to others for slowing nephropathy progression based on outcomes [32]. Each class will be briefly summarized and a general approach to achieving BP goal will be presented at the end of the chapter

Renin-angiotensin aldosterone system blockade

Antihypertensive agents that block the renin angiotensin-aldosterone system (RAAS) including angiotensin converting enzyme (ACE) inhibitors and angiotensin receptor blockers (ARBs) reduce the rate of both urinary albumin excretion and decline in kidney function. A summary of all such trials and effects on kidney disease progression and change in proteinuria are provided in Table 4.2.

While all antihypertensive agents reduce BP and slow CKD progression, no regimen is more efficacious in reducing proteinuria than one containing a RAAS blocker. ACE inhibitors and ARBs help prevent glomerulosclerosis in a manner that is independent of BP or glycemic control. This fact is supported by studies in normotensive patients with type 2 DM and microalbuminuria in whom the ACE inhibitor enalapril decreased the rate of progression to overt proteinuria (42% versus 12% in group receiving enalapril) [33].

Multiple clinical trials have examined the benefit of ACE inhibitors and ARBs in advanced stage proteinuric diabetic and hypertensive nephropathy. The benefit of these agents on slowing nephropathy progression was initially shown in a trial of 409 type I diabetics with overt nephropathy (albuminuria >500 mg/day) and mild renal insufficiency (serum creatinine <2.5 mg/dl) assigned to treatment with either captopril or placebo. After 3 years, the captopril treatment arm showed a 48% decrease in doubling of serum creatinine and a 30%

Table 4.2 Clinical trials and renal outcomes based on proteinuria reduction at six months.

Increased time to dialysis	*No change in time to dialysis*
(30–35% proteinuria reduction) Captopril Trial [35] AASK Trial [28] RENAAL [39] IDNT [40]	*(NO proteinuria reduction)* DHPCCB arm-IDNT DHPCCB arm-AASK
AASK = African American Study of Kidney Disease and Hypertension; IDNT = Irbesartan in Diabetic Nephropathy Trial; RENAAL = Reduction of Endpoints in NIDDM with the Angiotensin II Antagonist Losartan.	

decrease in albuminuria independent of BP control [34, 35]. Likewise, the Ramipril Efficacy In Nephropathy (REIN) trial showed decreased proteinuria and preserved kidney function in non-diabetic patients with kidney disease treated with an ACE inhibitor [36]. In this trial, patients with an average serum creatinine of 2.4 mg/dl and 24-h urine protein excretion >3 g/day were assigned either to ramipril 5 mg or to placebo. The ramipril group showed a 55% decrease in the composite endpoint of median urine protein excretion, doubling of serum creatinine, and GFR decline.

Intervention with a RAAS blocker protects against the development of microalbuminuria in hypertensive type 2 diabetic patients; however, this is not necessarily tied to nephropathy prevention or cardiovascular outcome. This was studied in the Bergamo Nephrologic Diabetes Mellitus Complications Trial (BENEDICT) [37]. In this trial, 1204 patients with hypertension and type 2 diabetes and normal urine albumin excretion were randomized to therapy with one of the following: the non-dihydropyridine calcium channel blocker verapamil, the ACE inhibitor trandolapril, a combination of verapamil and trandolapril, or placebo. After a median follow-up of 3.6 years, the onset of microalbuminuria was significantly lower in the subjects treated with trandolapril or the combination compared to the subjects receiving either verapamil or placebo.

ACE inhibitors and ARBs provide similar cardiovascular and renal protection in patients with diabetic and hypertensive nephropathy. This was supported by the Diabetics Exposed to Telmisartan and Enalapril Study [38], which compared the effects of enalapril and telmisartan in 250 patients with type 2 DM, hypertension and urine albumin excretion (UAE) between 11–999 µg/min. After 2 years, both agents showed similar effects on changes in GFR, UAE and serum creatinine levels.

The two major outcome trials that have evaluated the effect of ARBs on kidney disease progression in type 2 DM are the RENAAL trial [39] and the Irbesartan in Diabetic Nephropathy Trial (IDNT) [40]. The RENAAL trial randomized 1513 patients with type 2 DM who had a mean creatinine of 1.9 mg/dl and a median albumin to creatinine ratio of 1237 mg/g to either the ARB losartan or placebo, both in the addition to conventional antihypertensive treatment (but not ACE inhibitors). After 3.4 years, losartan reduced the primary endpoint of doubling of creatinine, progression to ESRD, or death by 16%. At the same time, a 35% reduction of albumin-creatinine ratio and a 15% decrease in loss of estimated creatinine clearance was seen in the losartan therapy group. This study concluded that renoprotection from ARB therapy was not related to BP but rather to the reduction in proteinuria.

In the IDNT 1715 patients with type 2 DM with a mean creatinine of 1.7 mg/dl and median urinary protein excretion of 2900 mg/day were randomized to irbesartan (300 mg), amlodipine (10 mg) or placebo in addition to conventional therapy (ACE inhibitors were not permitted). After a mean follow-up of 2.6 years, proteinuria decreased by 33% in the irbesartan group versus 6% in the amlodipine and 10% in the placebo group. There was also a 20% and 23% reduction of doubling of baseline creatinine, onset of ESRD or death in the irbesartan group when compared to the placebo and amlodipine groups, respectively.

The combined use of high-dose ACE inhibitors and ARBs can further reduce proteinuria by about 20–25% when compared to either ACE inhibitors or ARB monotherapy [41, 42]. The effect of further proteinuria reduction with combination ACE inhibitor and ARB therapy on kidney disease progression is unknown. The Combination Treatment of Angiotensin Receptor Blocker and Angiotensin Converting Enzyme Inhibitor in Non-diabetic Renal Disease (COOPERATE) trial, the only appropriately powered trial that evaluated dual blockade on non-diabetic kidney disease progression attempted to answer this question; however, the many data discrepancies in this study seriously limited its validity for drawing any conclusions on this issue [42, 43].

Renin inhibitors

Aliskiren was approved for the treatment of hypertension in 2007 and is the only clinically available renin inhibitor [44]. It represents a new class of agents in the manner by which it blocks the RAAS in that it specifically inhibits renin activity and thereby decreases angiotensin II levels and to a degree aldosterone. There appears to be an incremental benefit for BP reduction when aliskiren is combined with the ARB valsartan [45]; however, this additivity for BP reduction was not demonstrated when aliskiren was used as part of dual blockade with the ARB losartan in the Aliskiren in the Evaluation of proteinuria in Diabetes (AVOID) trial [46]. This was a randomized double-blind study involving 599 patients. Subjects enrolled in this study entered into a 3-month open label period where any previously administered drug that interfered with the RAAS was discontinued except β-blockers. Treatment was initiated with 100 mg of losartan in all participants and then patients were randomly assigned to either aliskiren (150 mg for 3 months titrated to 300 mg for next 3 months) or placebo for total of 6 months of therapy. The primary outcome was reduction in urinary albumin:creatinine (UACR). A reduction of 20% in UACR was observed in the aliskiren group when compared to placebo. About twice as many patients who received aliskiren had a >50% reduction in albuminuria compared to those receiving placebo.This trial suggested that aliskiren might have a renoprotective effect that is independent of its BP-lowering effect in patients with hypertension, type 2 DM, and nephropathy.

Perceived and real limitations to use of RAAS blockade

RAAS blockade related elevations in serum creatinine levels are well documented among those with renal insufficiency and renal arterial disease and is responsible for the reluctance of physicians to use RAAS blockade therapy in patients when creatinine values are nominally elevated (e.g. serum creatinine >1.4 mg/dl). The reason for this rise in creatinine with RAAS blockade is most often concurrent volume depletion or a low cardiac output state [32, 47]. The drop in BP in patients with renal dysfunction as well a change in efferent arteriolar tone reduces glomerular hydrostatic pressure leading to a small and limited decrease in GFR and ultimately a rise in serum creatinine. In general, at serum creatinine values of <3 mg/dl and age <65 years, a 30% to 35% increase in serum creatinine from baseline is acceptable within the first 3–4 months of RAAS blockade [13, 32, 47]. This change in serum creatinine usually stabilizes within 2–3 months. However, if an elevation in creatinine is more than 30–35 % and continues to rise, then the patient should be considered to be chronically volume depleted or to have bilateral renal artery stenosis [32, 47]. A rise in serum creatinine values with RAAS blockade may, however, be a marker of renoprotection. In that regard, a review of two independent studies found that an early elevation in serum creatinine in the absence of hyperkalemia translated into an overall slower rate of renal functional decline (Figure 4.1).

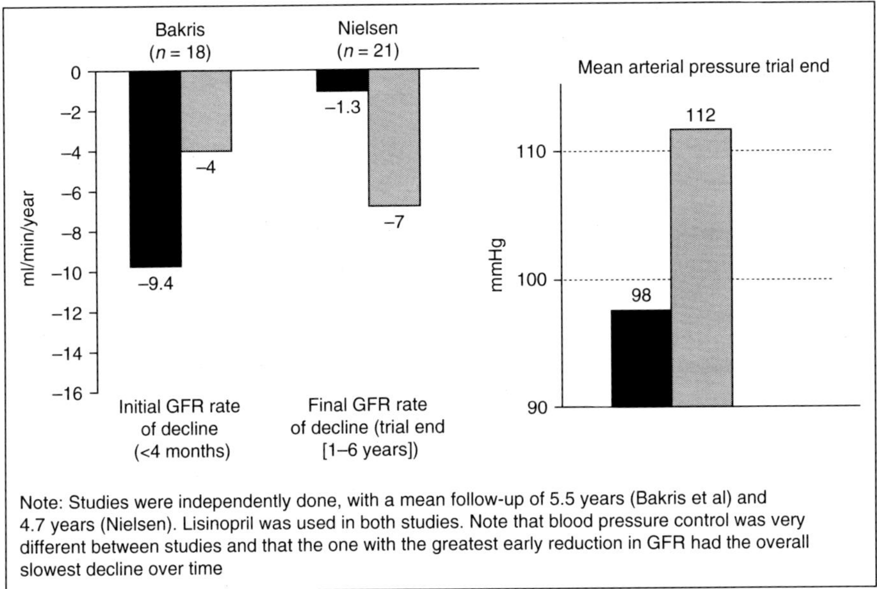

Figure 4.1 Early and late changes in the annual rate of GFR decline (adapted with permission from [47]).

Another common problem encountered with ACE inhibitors and ARBs that results in their discontinuation is hyperkalemia. Given the cardiovascular and renal benefits of these agents, they should only be discontinued if serum potassium rises to levels >5.7 mEq/l with all other etiologies of hyperkalemia (i.e. non-steroidal anti-inflammatory drugs [NSAIDs], high potassium diet, salt substitutes) having been eliminated [47, 48].

Diuretics

Thiazide diuretics are effective in lowering BP and reducing cardiovascular mortality [49]. However, as most patients with hypertensive nephropathy have reduced kidney function (i.e. GFR ≤40–50 ml/min) some thiazide diuretics such as hydrochlorothiazide are not as effective. Chlorthalidone, however, is quite effective for BP lowering and natriuresis [50]. For patients with an eGFR <50 ml/min, thiazide diuretics may not be effective and more potent loop diuretics like furosemide, twice daily, or torsemide are preferred.

Recent data demonstrate that aldosterone-receptor blockers in low doses can decrease proteinuria [51]. This is true for all aldosterone receptor blockers used either alone or in combination with an ACE inhibitor or ARB [52–54]. In that regard, spironolactone was studied in 59 patients with type 2 DM who were already on an ACE inhibitor or an ARB and compared to placebo [55]. The results showed a 40% decrease in the urine albumin to creatinine ratio in the spironolactone group when compared to placebo. However, patients on this combination should be monitored for hyperkalemia and should be instructed to follow a low potassium diet, and to avoid NSAIDs and other agents that may cause hyperkalemia.

Calcium channel blockers

Both dihydropyridine and non-dihydropyridine calcium channel blockers (CCBs) are effective in lowering BP but only non-dihydropyridine CCBs (diltiazem and verapamil) have demonstrated significant antiproteinuric effects in hypertensive patients with DM and proteinuria [56]. In previous studies of patients with overt proteinuric nephropathy, non-dihydropyridine CCBs reduced proteinuria and the rate of decline in creatinine clearance [57]. Differences in the renal effects between these subclasses of CCBs relates to impairment in renal autoregulation and glomerular permeability produced by dihydropyridine CCBs [58, 59]. Specifically, dihydropyridine CCBs disable the ability of the afferent arteriole to constrict and dampen intraglomerular pressure if systemic pressure is increased. Hence, intraglomerular pressure increases in parallel to systemic pressure. Thus, use of these agents mandates a lower systemic pressure to yield a similar level of intraglomerular pressure seen with agents that don't interfere with autoregulation [60]. This increases intraglomerular pressure leads to increases in membrane permeability to albumin [57, 61]. On the other hand, non-dihydropyridine CCBs only partially interfere with glomerular autoregulation, leaving the afferent arteriole partially functional to constrict in response to increases in systemic pressure and reduce glomerular permeability to a greater extent [60, 62].

These differences in CCBs are only relevant in people with advanced proteinuric kidney disease defined as >300 mg/day of urinary protein excretion but not in those with microalbuminuria or early stage kidney disease [63]. Hence, the current evidence suggests that although dihydropyridine CCBs are effective in lowering BP in patients with CKD, they should not be used as monotherapy in diabetic or non-diabetic kidney disease with proteinuria, but always in combination with an ACE inhibitor or an ARB, if BP is not adequately controlled [32].

Beta-blockers

There is no direct evidence that conventional early generation β-blockers slow CKD progression or offer additional antiproteinuric effects beyond what might be anticipated with BP reduction [64]. Once daily sustained-release metoprolol has been shown to slow nephropathy progression and reduce albuminuria in the AASK trial, but the observed effects were not as significant as with the ACE inhibitor ramipril [28].

The newer vasodilating β-blockers, such as carvedilol, may differ from early generation β-blockers such as metoprolol. The Glycemic Effects in Diabetes Mellitus Carvedilol-Metoprolol Comparison in Hypertensives (GEMINI) trial compared carvedilol to metoprolol in type 2 diabetics with hypertension who were already on RAAS blockade [65]. There was a 16% reduction in microalbuminuria in the carvedilol group and 47% fewer patients with normoalbuminuria progressed to microalbuminuria on carvedilol when compared to subjects in the metoprolol group [66].

There are sparse data on cardiovascular outcomes with β-blockers in advanced nephropathy, therefore, the effective use of these compounds is based on inference for cardiovascular outcomes and demonstrated effect for BP reduction in advanced nephropathy [67]. It would seem that β-blockers would be helpful as third or fourth line therapy to lower BP in patients with CKD. These agents are also acceptable in CKD patients with significant heart failure or coronary artery disease.

General approach to achieve BP goals in nephropathy

The basic paradigm to achieve BP goals in people with hypertensive CKD has not changed appreciably from that suggested in JNC-7 and the Kidney Disease Outcome Quality Initiative (KDOQI) guidelines [13, 32]. Blockers of the RAAS system are still recommended as initial agents for BP lowering along with a second agent, usually a CCB or thiazide-like diuretic, if >20/10 mmHg above the guideline goal BP of <130/80 mmHg. Since no difference in cardiovascular outcomes has been noted between antihypertensive agents if BP is appropriately lowered [49], this approach mitigates against worsening of metabolic control [68]. Specifically, achieving a blood pressure target with agents that do not worsen glucose toler-

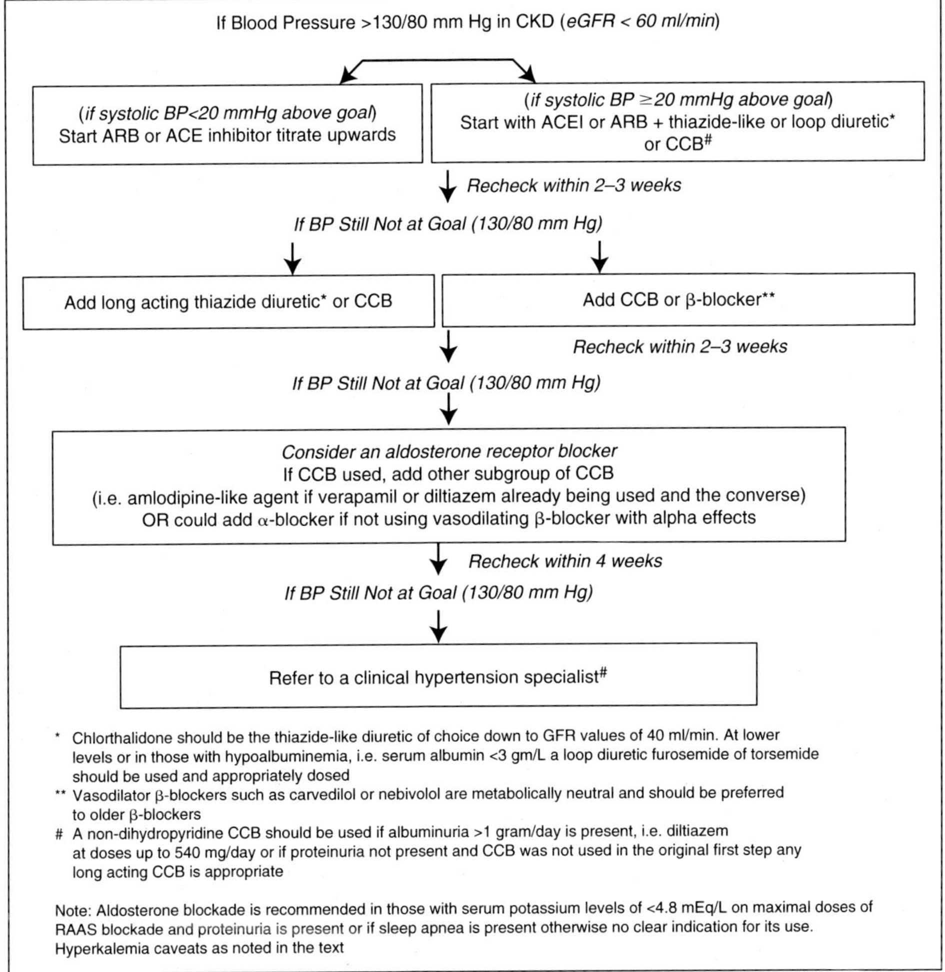

Figure 4.2 Algorithm for achieving blood pressure goal in hypertensive CKD (adapted with permission from [69, 70]).

ance or produce lipid abnormalities would be preferred to achieving the same targets with agents that have such side-effects.

A recommended approach to achieve BP goal and optimize cardiovascular and renal protection in the setting of nephropathy is summarized in Figure 4.2 [69, 70]. Lifestyle changes should have a central role in helping to manage hypertension in all patients with a BP ≥130/80 mmHg. These include weight loss, increase in physical exercise, reduction of alcohol intake, smoking cessation, and, perhaps most importantly, low sodium intake, which should be encouraged through appropriate dietary counseling (Table 4.1).

Whether choosing an ACE inhibitor or an ARB, dosage should be titrated to the highest level necessary for BP to reach goal. If an ACE inhibitor is started and the side-effect of cough appears, treatment should be changed to an appropriate dose of an ARB. If, within one month after monotherapy titration the BP goal is not achieved, then a long acting CCB or thiazide-like diuretic (e.g. 12.5 mg of chlorthalidone) should be added. In the case of a patient with nephropathy and eGFR <50 ml/min, the thiazide diuretic should be replaced by a loop diuretic in adequate doses (once daily torsemide or twice daily furosemide or bumetanide). Note chlorthalidone can be used in such patients down to a GFR of 40 ml/min if not sometimes lower GFR values. If proteinuria >300 mg/day is present, a non-dihydropyridine CCB is preferred over a dihydropyridine CCB in order to maximally reduce proteinuria [32, 57]. In addition, minimization of the number of pills of antihypertensive drugs improves patient adherence and effectiveness of lowering BP [71, 72]. Thus, conversion of the full combination treatment to a fixed dose combination of RAAS blocker/diuretic or RAAS blocker/CCB should be given strong consideration.

If after 2 to 4 weeks of adding a diuretic or CCB BP is still not at goal, consider either titrating to 25 mg/day of chlorthalidone or maximum tolerated dose of CCB. As noted in Figure 4.1, this combination of medications will ensure that target BP is achieved in the majority of cases. However, in at least of 30% of the remaining cases a fourth and possibly a fifth agent will be needed [9]. Under these circumstances, a β-blocker is useful. Moreover, a vasodilating β-blocker is generally better tolerated and can be metabolically neutral compared to vasoconstricting agents [68]. Beta-blockers are especially useful in people with elevated pulse rates and a β-blocker should be considered for BP control if the pulse rate is >84 beats per minute on at least two separate antihypertensive medications. Alternatively, combination of a non-dihydropyridine CCB (verapamil or diltiazem) in moderate to high doses with a dihydropyridine CCB has been shown to have clear additive effects on BP reduction [73] and will help achieve goal BP. Finally, consideration should be given to use of a combination of maximal dose ACE inhibitor or ARB with an aldosterone antagonist to reduce urine albumin excretion in patients with more than one gram of proteinuria not responding to effective BP control [53]. As previously discussed, monitoring for hyperkalemia should occur and this combination not used when baseline potassium on a RAAS blocker is at or above 4.8 mEq/l.

SUMMARY

Hypertensive kidney disease can only be diagnosed with a blood test to assess kidney function, especially a serum creatinine. This is then placed into an equation that is available in most commercial labs that can produce an estimated glomerular filtration rate (eGFR). An eGFR <60 ml/min is consistent with a diagnosis of chronic kidney disease. Additionally, urine albumin needs to be assessed as this has prognostic implications both for nephropathy progression and cardiovascular risk. Presence of a urine albumin of >30 mg/day but <300 mg day indicates increased cardiovascular risk; ≥300 mg/day of albumin indicates the presence of kidney disease and a higher risk for CKD progression unless reduced.

The key to preservation of kidney function is appropriate blood pressure control to levels below 140/90 mmHg and, if albuminuria is present in excess of 300 mg/day, <130/80 mmHg. A blocker of the renin-angiotensin system must be part of the therapeutic regimen along with either a calcium antagonist or diuretic, if needed to achieve the blood pressure goal. In most cases of established kidney disease, three or even four drugs will be needed to reduce blood pressure to appropriate levels. Early increases in serum creatinine (within 2–4 months of an ACE inhibitor or ARB) of about 30% are acceptable in the absence of hyperkalemia and correlate with better long-term renal outcomes.

REFERENCES

1. Schoolwerth AC, Engelgau MM, Hostetter TH *et al*. Chronic kidney disease: a public health problem that needs a public health action plan. *Prev Chronic Dis* 2006; 3:A57.
2. Coresh J, Selvin E, Stevens LA *et al*. Prevalence of chronic kidney disease in the United States. *JAMA* 2007; 298:2038–2047.

3. KDOQI Clinical Practice Guidelines and Clinical Practice Recommendations for Diabetes and Chronic Kidney Disease. *Am J Kidney Dis* 2007; 49:S12–S154.

4. Buckalew VM Jr, Berg RL, Wang SR, Porush JG, Rauch S, Schulman G. Prevalence of hypertension in 1,795 subjects with chronic renal disease: the modification of diet in renal disease study baseline cohort. Modification of Diet in Renal Disease Study Group. *Am J Kidney Dis* 1996; 28:811–821.

5. Weir MR. The role of combination antihypertensive therapy in the prevention and treatment of chronic kidney disease. *Am J Hypertens* 2005; 18:100S–105S.

6. Rao MV, Qiu Y, Wang C, Bakris G. Hypertension and CKD: Kidney Early Evaluation Program (KEEP) and National Health and Nutrition Examination Survey (NHANES), 1999–2004. *Am J Kidney Dis* 2008; 51:S30–S37.

7. Bakris GL. Should a lower blood pressure goal and albuminuria reduction be mandated to slow hypertensive nephropathy? *Curr Hypertens Rep* 2008; 10:387–388.

8. Calhoun DA, Zaman MA, Nishizaka MK. Resistant hypertension. *Curr Hypertens Rep* 2002; 4:221–228.

9. Sarafidis PA, Bakris GL. Resistant hypertension: an overview of evaluation and treatment. *J Am Coll Cardiol* 2008; 52:1749–1757.

10. Khosla N, Sarafidis PA, Bakris GL. Microalbuminuria. *Clin Lab Med* 2006; 26:635–653, vi–vii. Review.

11. Bakris GL. *Microalbuminuria: Marker of Kidney and Cardiovascular Disease*, 2nd edition. Current Medicine Group, London, 2007.

12. Mancia G, De BG, Dominiczak A *et al.* 2007 Guidelines for the Management of Arterial Hypertension: The Task Force for the Management of Arterial Hypertension of the European Society of Hypertension (ESH) and of the European Society of Cardiology (ESC). *J Hypertens* 2007; 25:1105–1187.

13. Chobanian AV, Bakris GL, Black HR *et al.* The seventh report of the Joint National Committee on Prevention, Detection, Evaluation, and Treatment of High Blood Pressure: the JNC-7 report. *JAMA* 2003; 289:2560–2572.

14. Gerstein HC, Mann JF, Yi Q *et al.* Albuminuria and risk of cardiovascular events, death, and heart failure in diabetic and nondiabetic individuals. *JAMA* 2001; 286:421–426.

15. Kistorp C, Raymond I, Pedersen F, Gustafsson F, Faber J, Hildebrandt P. N-terminal pro-brain natriuretic peptide, C-reactive protein, and urinary albumin levels as predictors of mortality and cardiovascular events in older adults. *JAMA* 2005; 293:1609–1616.

16. Jerums G, Panagiotopoulos S, Premaratne E, Power DA, MacIsaac RJ. Lowering of proteinuria in response to antihypertensive therapy predicts improved renal function in late but not in early diabetic nephropathy: a pooled analysis. *Am J Nephrol* 2008; 28:614–627.

17. Estacio RO, Jeffers BW, Gifford N, Schrier RW. Effect of blood pressure control on diabetic microvascular complications in patients with hypertension and type 2 diabetes. *Diabetes Care* 2000; 23:B54–B64.

18. Schrier RW, Estacio RO, Mehler PS, Hiatt WR. Appropriate blood pressure control in hypertensive and normotensive type 2 diabetes mellitus: a summary of the ABCD trial. *Nat Clin Pract Nephrol* 2007; 3:428–438.

19. Eijkelkamp WB, Zhang Z, Remuzzi G *et al.* Albuminuria is a target for renoprotective therapy independent from blood pressure in patients with type 2 diabetic nephropathy: post hoc analysis from the Reduction of Endpoints in NIDDM with the Angiotensin II Antagonist Losartan (RENAAL) trial. *J Am Soc Nephrol* 2007; 18:1540–1546.

20. Lea J, Greene T, Hebert L *et al.* The relationship between magnitude of proteinuria reduction and risk of end-stage renal disease: results of the African American study of kidney disease and hypertension. *Arch Intern Med* 2005; 165:947–953.

21. Atkins RC, Briganti EM, Lewis JB *et al.* Proteinuria reduction and progression to renal failure in patients with type 2 diabetes mellitus and overt nephropathy. *Am J Kidney Dis* 2005; 45:281–287.

22. Tight blood pressure control and risk of macrovascular and microvascular complications in type 2 diabetes: UKPDS 38. UK Prospective Diabetes Study Group. *BMJ* 1998; 317:703–713.

23. Hansson L, Zanchetti A, Carruthers SG *et al.* Effects of intensive blood-pressure lowering and low-dose aspirin in patients with hypertension: principal results of the Hypertension Optimal Treatment (HOT) randomised trial. HOT Study Group. *Lancet* 1998; 351:1755–1762.

24. Buse JB, Bigger JT, Byington RP *et al.* Action to Control Cardiovascular Risk in Diabetes (ACCORD) trial: design and methods. *Am J Cardiol* 2007; 99:21i–33i.

25. Peterson JC, Adler S, Burkart JM *et al.* Blood pressure control, proteinuria, and the progression of renal disease. The Modification of Diet in Renal Disease Study. *Ann Intern Med* 1995; 123:754–762.

26. Klahr S, Levey AS, Beck GJ *et al*. The effects of dietary protein restriction and blood-pressure control on the progression of chronic renal disease. Modification of Diet in Renal Disease Study Group. *N Engl J Med* 1994; 330:877–884.

27. Sarnak MJ, Greene T, Wang X *et al*. The effect of a lower target blood pressure on the progression of kidney disease: long-term follow-up of the modification of diet in renal disease study. *Ann Intern Med* 2005; 142:342–351.

28. Wright JT Jr, Bakris G, Greene T *et al*. Effect of blood pressure lowering and antihypertensive drug class on progression of hypertensive kidney disease: results from the AASK trial. *JAMA* 2002; 288:2421–2431.

29. Appel LJ, Wright JT Jr, Greene T *et al*. Long-term effects of renin-angiotensin system-blocking therapy and a low blood pressure goal on progression of hypertensive chronic kidney disease in African Americans. *Arch Intern Med* 2008; 168:832–839.

30. Jafar TH, Schmid CH, Stark PC *et al*. The rate of progression of renal disease may not be slower in women compared with men: a patient-level meta-analysis. *Nephrol Dial Transplant* 2003; 18:2047–2053.

31. Fogo A, Breyer JA, Smith MC *et al*. Accuracy of the diagnosis of hypertensive nephrosclerosis in African Americans: a report from the African American Study of Kidney Disease (AASK) Trial. AASK Pilot Study Investigators. *Kidney Int* 1997; 51:244–252.

32. KDOQI clinical practice guidelines on hypertension and antihypertensive agents in chronic kidney disease. *Am J Kidney Dis* 2004; 43:S1–S290.

33. Ravid M, Lang R, Rachmani R, Lishner M. Long-term renoprotective effect of angiotensin-converting enzyme inhibition in non-insulin-dependent diabetes mellitus. A 7-year follow-up study. *Arch Intern Med* 1996; 156:286–289.

34. Wilmer WA, Hebert LA, Lewis EJ *et al*. Remission of nephrotic syndrome in type 1 diabetes: long-term follow-up of patients in the Captopril Study. *Am J Kidney Dis* 1999; 34:308–314.

35. Lewis EJ, Hunsicker LG, Bain RP, Rohde RD. The effect of angiotensin-converting-enzyme inhibition on diabetic nephropathy. The Collaborative Study Group. *N Engl J Med* 1993; 329:1456–1462.

36. Randomised placebo-controlled trial of effect of ramipril on decline in glomerular filtration rate and risk of terminal renal failure in proteinuric, non-diabetic nephropathy. The GISEN Group (Gruppo Italiano di Studi Epidemiologici in Nefrologia). *Lancet* 1997; 349:1857–1863.

37. Ruggenenti P, Fassi A, Ilieva AP *et al*. Preventing microalbuminuria in type 2 diabetes. *N Engl J Med* 2004; 351:1941–1951.

38. Barnett AH, Bain SC, Bouter P *et al*. Angiotensin-receptor blockade versus converting-enzyme inhibition in type 2 diabetes and nephropathy. *N Engl J Med* 2004; 351:1952–1961.

39. Brenner BM, Cooper ME, de Zeeuw D *et al*. Effects of losartan on renal and cardiovascular outcomes in patients with type 2 diabetes and nephropathy. *N Engl J Med* 2001; 345:861–869.

40. Lewis EJ, Hunsicker LG, Clarke WR *et al*. Renoprotective effect of the angiotensin-receptor antagonist irbesartan in patients with nephropathy due to type 2 diabetes. *N Engl J Med* 2001; 345:851–860.

41. Casas JP, Chua W, Loukogeorgakis S *et al*. Effect of inhibitors of the renin-angiotensin system and other antihypertensive drugs on renal outcomes: systematic review and meta-analysis. *Lancet* 2005; 366:2026–2033.

42. Kunz R, Friedrich C, Wolbers M, Mann JF. Meta-analysis: effect of monotherapy and combination therapy with inhibitors of the renin angiotensin system on proteinuria in renal disease. *Ann Intern Med* 2008; 148:30–48.

43. Bidani A. Controversy about COOPERATE ABPM trial data. *Am J Nephrol* 2006; 26:629–632.

44. Gradman AH, Schmieder RE, Lins RL, Nussberger J, Chiang Y, Bedigian MP. Aliskiren, a novel orally effective renin inhibitor, provides dose-dependent antihypertensive efficacy and placebo-like tolerability in hypertensive patients. *Circulation* 2005; 111:1012–1018.

45. Oparil S, Yarows SA, Patel S, Fang H, Zhang J, Satlin A. Efficacy and safety of combined use of aliskiren and valsartan in patients with hypertension: a randomised, double-blind trial. *Lancet* 2007; 370:221–229.

46. Parving HH, Persson F, Lewis JB, Lewis EJ, Hollenberg NK. Aliskiren combined with losartan in type 2 diabetes and nephropathy. *N Engl J Med* 2008; 358:2433–2446.

47. Bakris GL, Weir MR. Angiotensin-converting enzyme inhibitor-associated elevations in serum creatinine: is this a cause for concern? *Arch Intern Med* 2000; 160:685–693.

48. Pitt B, Bakris G, Ruilope LM, DiCarlo L, Mukherjee R. Serum potassium and clinical outcomes in the Eplerenone Post-Acute Myocardial Infarction Heart Failure Efficacy and Survival Study (EPHESUS). *Circulation* 2008; 118:1643–1650.

49. Turnbull F, Neal B, Ninomiya T *et al.* Effects of different regimens to lower blood pressure on major cardiovascular events in older and younger adults: meta-analysis of randomised trials. *BMJ* 2008; 336:1121–1123.
50. Carter BL, Ernst ME, Cohen JD. Hydrochlorothiazide versus chlorthalidone: evidence supporting their interchangeability. *Hypertension* 2004; 43:4–9.
51. Rachmani R, Slavachevsky I, Amit M *et al.* The effect of spironolactone, cilazapril and their combination on albuminuria in patients with hypertension and diabetic nephropathy is independent of blood pressure reduction: a randomized controlled study. *Diabet Med* 2004; 21:471–475.
52. van den Meiracker AH, Baggen RG, Pauli S *et al.* Spironolactone in type 2 diabetic nephropathy: effects on proteinuria, blood pressure and renal function. *J Hypertens* 2006; 24:2285–2292.
53. Bomback AS, Kshirsagar AV, Amamoo MA, Klemmer PJ. Change in proteinuria after adding aldosterone blockers to ACE inhibitors or angiotensin receptor blockers in CKD: a systematic review. *Am J Kidney Dis* 2008; 51:199–211.
54. Epstein M, Williams GH, Weinberger M *et al.* Selective aldosterone blockade with eplerenone reduces albuminuria in patients with type 2 diabetes. *Clin J Am Soc Nephrol* 2006; 1:940–951.
55. Han SY, Kim CH, Kim HS *et al.* Spironolactone prevents diabetic nephropathy through an anti-inflammatory mechanism in type 2 diabetic rats. *J Am Soc Nephrol* 2006; 17:1362–1372.
56. Bohlen L, de Courten M, Weidmann P. Comparative study of the effect of ACE-inhibitors and other antihypertensive agents on proteinuria in diabetic patients. *Am J Hypertens* 1994; 7:84S–92S.
57. Bakris GL, Weir MR, Secic M, Campbell B, Weis-McNulty A. Differential effects of calcium antagonist subclasses on markers of nephropathy progression. *Kidney Int* 2004; 65:1991–2002.
58. Griffin KA, Hacioglu R, bu-Amarah I, Loutzenhiser R, Williamson GA, Bidani AK. Effects of calcium channel blockers on "dynamic" and "steady-state step" renal autoregulation. *Am J Physiol Renal Physiol* 2004; 286:F1136–F1143.
59. Smith AC, Toto R, Bakris GL. Differential effects of calcium channel blockers on size selectivity of proteinuria in diabetic glomerulopathy. *Kidney Int* 1998; 54:889–896.
60. Kvam FI, Ofstad J, Iversen BM. Effects of antihypertensive drugs on autoregulation of RBF and glomerular capillary pressure in SHR. *Am J Physiol* 1998; 275:F576–F584.
61. Nathan S, Pepine CJ, Bakris GL. Calcium antagonists: effects on cardio-renal risk in hypertensive patients. *Hypertension* 2005; 46:637–642.
62. Griffin KA, Picken MM, Bakris GL, Bidani AK. Class differences in the effects of calcium channel blockers in the rat remnant kidney model. *Kidney Int* 1999; 55:1849–1860.
63. Hart P, Bakris GL. Calcium antagonists: do they equally protect against kidney injury? *Kidney Int* 2008; 73:795–796.
64. Efficacy of atenolol and captopril in reducing risk of macrovascular and microvascular complications in type 2 diabetes: UKPDS 39. UK Prospective Diabetes Study Group. *BMJ* 1998; 317:713–720.
65. Bakris GL, Fonseca V, Katholi RE *et al.* Metabolic effects of carvedilol vs metoprolol in patients with type 2 diabetes mellitus and hypertension: a randomized controlled trial. *JAMA* 2004; 292:2227–2236.
66. Bakris GL, Fonseca V, Katholi RE *et al.* Differential effects of beta-blockers on albuminuria in patients with type 2 diabetes. *Hypertension* 2005; 46:1309–1315.
67. Bakris GL, Hart P, Ritz E. Beta blockers in the management of chronic kidney disease. *Kidney Int* 2006; 70:1905–1913.
68. Sarafidis PA, McFarlane SI, Bakris GL. Antihypertensive agents, insulin sensitivity, and new-onset diabetes. *Curr Diab Rep* 2007; 7:191–199.
69. Bakris GL, Sowers JR. ASH position paper: treatment of hypertension in patients with diabetes – an update. *J Clin Hypertens (Greenwich)* 2008; 10:707–713; discussion 714–715.
70. Ruilope L, Kjeldsen SE, de la Sierra A *et al.* The kidney and cardiovascular risk – implications for management: a consensus statement from the European Society of Hypertension. *Blood Press* 2007; 16:72–79.
71. Bangalore S, Kamalakkannan G, Parkar S, Messerli FH. Fixed-dose combinations improve medication compliance: a meta-analysis. *Am J Med* 2007; 120:713–719.
72. Gerbino PP, Shoheiber O. Adherence patterns among patients treated with fixed-dose combination versus separate antihypertensive agents. *Am J Health Syst Pharm* 2007; 64:1279–1283.
73. Saseen JJ, Carter BL, Brown TE, Elliott WJ, Black HR. Comparison of nifedipine alone and with diltiazem or verapamil in hypertension. *Hypertension* 1996; 28:109–114.

5

How low should systolic and diastolic blood pressure be?

N. Karakala, D. S. Hanes, M. R. Weir

BACKGROUND

Hypertension is a major medical and public health concern throughout the world. Data from the National Health and Nutrition Examination Survey (NHANES) has indicated that 50 million or more Americans have high blood pressure that will need some form of intervention [1]. Worldwide prevalence estimates for hypertension may be as high as 1 billion individuals, and approximately 7.1 million deaths per year may be attributed to hypertension [2]. With improving awareness among the population and more intense screening and treatment by physicians there has been a significant improvement in the percentage of people optimally treated for hypertension.

Hypertension is a life-long, progressive, asymptomatic disease that affects individuals at a variable rate depending on their age, genetic background, and interaction with the environment; hence the need for longitudinal screening and monitoring. Hypertension is dynamic condition: a normotensive person can develop hypertension at anytime in the future, and by the age of 55 years will have a 90% lifetime risk of subsequently developing hypertension. For this reason all previously normotensive patients should be actively screened with increasing age. Moreover, the risk of coronary vascular disease in hypertensive patients is consistent, graded and independent of other risk factors. The presence of other risk factors like diabetes mellitus, age, smoking, kidney disease, and hyperlipidemia compound this risk. The World Health Organization reports that suboptimal BP is responsible for 62% of cerebrovascular disease and 49% of ischemic heart disease (IHD) with little variation between males and females [2]. Data from observational studies with more than 1 million individuals indicate that death from both IHD and stroke increases progressively as blood pressure (BP) rises above a systolic of 115 mmHg and diastolic of 75 mmHg. Follow-up from the Framingham Heart study reported an increased incidence of poor outcomes as BP rises, even within the normal range. This study examined the risk of cardiovascular (CV) disease at 10 years follow-up among subjects with high normal BP, which is defined as a

Nithin Karakala, MD, Internal Medicine Resident, St Agnes Hospital, Baltimore, Maryland, USA.

Donna S. Hanes, MD, Associate Professor of Medicine, Division of Nephrology, University of Maryland Hospital, Baltimore, Maryland, USA.

Matthew R. Weir, MD, Professor and Director, Division of Nephrology, University of Maryland School of Medicine, Baltimore, Maryland, USA.

systolic blood pressure (SBP) of 130–139 mmHg and a diastolic blood pressure (DBP) of 85–89 mmHg, and with normal BP defined as a SBP 120–129 mmHg and a DBP 80–84 mmHg. The hazard ratios for CV events for those with high normal BP values were 2.5 and 1.6 for women and men, respectively, compared to those with optimal BP values.. Patients with normal BP values also had an increase in the hazard ratio for a CV event compared with those having optimal BP. Based on these and other similar data , the JNC-7 added a new BP risk category called 'pre-hypertension' (SBP 120–139 mmHg, DBP 80–89 mmHg) [3].

It is proven beyond doubt that hypertension is a risk factor for cardiovascular disease (CVD), heart failure (HF), end-stage renal disease (ESRD) and stroke. The question of what is the optimal BP is one of great interest and the basis of numerous studies. Currently, comorbid conditions determine the optimal target BP, but the extent to which BP should be lowered beyond optimal values remains unanswered. Optimal BP values can be achieved with lifestyle modifications and/or pharmacotherapy, such as a low salt diet, exercise and smoking cessation contributing to the antihypertensive effects of medications. Lifestyle modifications often do not have a sustained effect on BP. This chapter will examine the evidence for lower BP targets. The choice, dose and combination of antihypertensive medications depend on a number of factors like age, race, comorbid conditions, tolerability, cost, and treatment adherence.

OPTIMAL BLOOD PRESSURE IN HIGH PULSE PRESSURE HYPERTENSION

The importance of BP as a determinant of CV risk and the benefit of treating hypertension is well established. It is important to determine which BP measures (SBP, DBP, pulse pressure [PP]) are more important in risk stratification and what is the optimal range for each when abnormal. The risk for CVD, stroke and renal disease depends on SBP, DBP, and PP in varying proportions. Previous studies described diastolic hypertension as the most important determinant of CVD risk, which has been recently challenged. Data from the Framingham study shows that DBP has a stronger correlation with CVD risk in individuals with hypertension who are less than about age 55 [3]. For individuals over the age of 55 years, CVD risk increases in tandem with rising SBPs and widening PPs more so than with isolated diastolic hypertension. Findings from several studies support the concept that CV events are more closely related to the pulsatile stress transmitted to stiff large arteries than to the steady flow/stress directed to the small arteries [4]. In older people the PP is a good measure of arterial stiffness, which is a key determinant of CVD risk. It is the aortic PP more so than the peripheral PP, that determines the CV risk. The difference in aortic and peripheral PP varies with age. In younger populations there still exists a significant difference in these two variables with the peripheral PP failing to closely correlate with aortic PP. In the young population, the diastolic and mean arterial pressures are similar in both the large and the small arteries. For this reason, diastolic BP becomes an important determinant of the CVD risk. But in older populations there is a smaller difference in aortic and peripheral PPs, which allows this measure to serve as a surrogate for hypertensive stress on the myocardium [5].

Domanski and colleagues evaluated the prognostic importance of systolic and diastolic BP and PP on CV mortality [6]. This study included men between the ages of 35 to 57 years divided into two groups (35 to 44 years and 45 to 57 years) to study effects of different parameters of BP as per different JNC-VI BP stratification groups (Figure 5.1). This study determined that SBP and DBP were stronger predictors of CV-related deaths than was PP. Of note, the higher the SBP the greater the CV risk in all age groups. For men in categories of high normal and stage 1 or stage 2–3 hypertension, the association of DBP and PP with CV disease related mortality varied with age. For men aged 35 to 44 years, elevation of both SBP and DBP carried an increased risk of CV disease. In contrast, in males aged 45 to 57 years, a higher CV risk was associated with either the discordant pattern of an elevated SBP

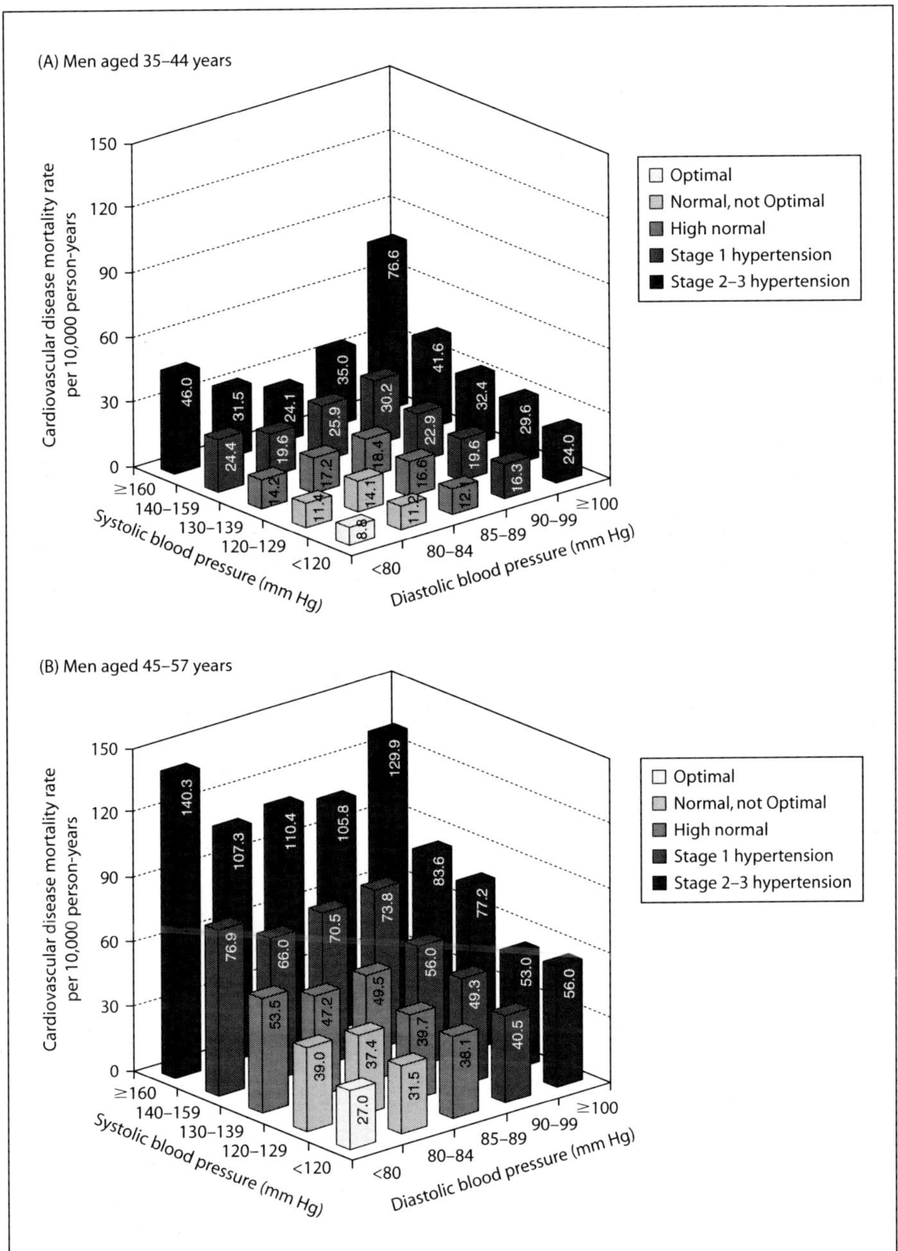

Figure 5.1 Age-adjusted cardiovascular disease mortality rate by systolic and diastolic blood pressure level used to define each JNC-VI stratum.

and a low DBP when DBP was below 80 mmHg (higher PP) or with the concordant pattern of both an elevated SBP and DBP. Cardiovascular disease related mortality risk was 28% higher for men with a SBP falling between 130 and 139 mmHg and a DBP below 80 mmHg vs. men with a SBP lower than 130 and a DBP of 85 to 89 mmHg. In the same age group, CV disease related mortality was 47% and 70 % higher for BPs (140–159/90–94 and SBP >160/95, respectively). This study shows that DBP and SBP together play a more important role than any one individual parameter.

The National Heath and Nutrition Survey II data [7] showed similar results although in a slightly different age group. For populations under 65 years of age, SBP was linearly related to all cause and CVD mortality for all DBP levels. The relationship of DBP and mortality in this age group was higher with DBPs above 80 mmHg, but there was no significant decrease in the relative risk below this BP level. In an older population age >65 years, SBP values showed a similar linear increase in risk, while diastolic blood pressure demonstrated a J-shaped relation for all cause and CVD mortality. For fixed DBP values, increasing SBP was associated with increased risk. For a fixed SBP, DBPs below 80 mmHg and above 90 mmHg were associated with an increased risk for CVD related mortality. Increasing PP secondary to elevated SBP was associated with an increased CVD risk. Similarly, increasing PP secondary to lower DBPs was also associated with an increased risk. Other studies failed to reproduce the J curve effect of DBP on CV risk [8]. The J curve phenomenon can be explained by the fact that the augmented systolic pressure causes left ventricular hypertrophy, which increases the systolic load and myocardial oxygen demand, and the low diastolic pressure causes peripheral runoff thereby causing decreased coronary perfusion and possible flow-dependent myocardial ischemia. It is not likely that purposeful reduction of SBP to a point that DBP is too low for coronary perfusion commonly occurs. More likely, the mortality in patients with low DBP is indicative of patients with a stiff aorta, wide PP and greater burden of atherosclerotic cardiovascular disease.

IS THERE A RISK OF LOWERING DIASTOLIC BLOOD PRESSURE TOO MUCH?

Several early trials indicated that lowering DBP too much could be detrimental. In a trial by Stewart on uncomplicated hypertension, patients whose DBP was lowered to <90 mmHg had five times the rate of myocardial infarction as those patients whose final DBP was 100 to 109 mmHg (Figure 5.2) [9]. Another study several years later reaffirmed the finding that in patients with evidence of cardiac ischemia at baseline, the optimal BP to minimize the risk of myocardial infarction was between 85 and 90 mmHg [10]. Treatment to a higher or lower DBP was associated with an increased risk of myocardial infarction. This phenomena has been termed the so called J-shaped curve. To date, this result has only been seen in those subjects with evidence of ischemic heart disease. Indeed, the speculation was that those patients with underlying ischemia could be "at risk" of over treatment with antihypertensive drugs. Because a rapid heart rate may be an important predictor of risk in patients with coronary artery disease [CAD], (whose coronary arteries are perfused during diastole), lowering DBP too far could prove detrimental. It is interesting to note that those studies that demonstrate a J-shaped curve frequently include patients with intercurrent heart disease.

The Hypertension Optimal Treatment (HOT) study was designed to specifically address the varied opinions concerning the J-shaped curve and mortality [8]. The study enrolled 18790 patients with a DBP of 100 to 115 mmHg. They were randomly assigned to one of three DBP groups: <90 mmHg, < 85 mmHg, and <80 mmHg. The SBP was reduced by 26 to 30 mmHg and DBP by 20 to 24 mmHg. At the end of the study, mean DBP differed by only 4 mmHg (85 to 81 mmHg) between the groups. There was a trend toward lower risk of myocardial infarction in the <85 mmHg and <80 mmHg, 25% and 28% respectively, than in the <90 mmHg target group despite more aggressive therapy. Moreover, up to 92% of patients were able to achieve DBP <90 mmHg. This study therefore dispelled the theory that aggressive antihypertensive therapy with multiple agents resulted in a J-curve in the absence of underlying heart disease.

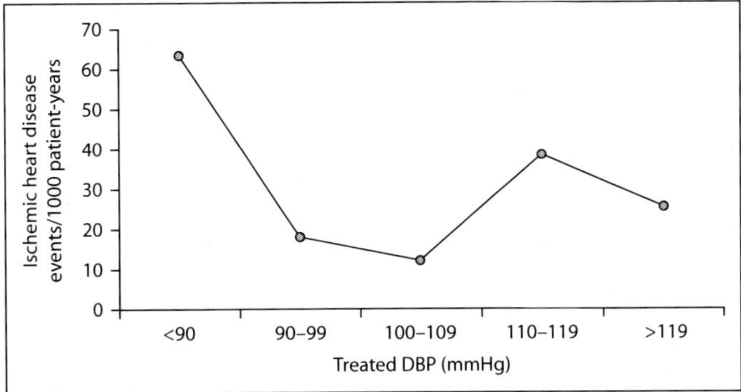

Figure 5.2 Rate of ischemic heart disease events as a function of treated diastolic blood pressure (DBP).

ANTIHYPERTENSIVES IN WIDE PULSE PRESSURE HYPERTENSION

In patients with an increased PP form of hypertension, either from isolated systolic hypertension or a discordant elevation in SBP with a low DBP, the goal of therapy is to decrease SBP with little or no effect on DBP. A large Veterans Affairs Cooperative Study examined the efficacy of six different classes of antihypertensive medications and their effect on PP. Of the studied drugs (clonidine, hydrochlorothiazide (HCTZ), atenolol, diltiazem SR, prazosin and captopril), clonidine and HCTZ had the greatest effect on PP. Patients randomized to clonidine or HCTZ achieved the goal PP of <55 mmHg more frequently than did those treated with either atenolol, diltiazem-SR, prazosin or captopril [11]. Patients taking clonidine had higher rates of adverse effects (fatigue, dizziness, sleepiness, and dry mouth) than was the case with the other drug classes [12]. Because of the ability of HCTZ to decrease PP better than most of the other drugs, combined with a low side-effect profile, it is a drug of choice in elderly patients with a high PP form of hypertension. Nitrates selectively decrease SBP over DBP but are not used as the first line treatment because of their well-known side-effects like headaches and orthostatic hypotension. *In vivo* rat studies show that the ACE inhibitor (perindopril) can decrease PP by preventing chronic collagen accumulation/deposition in the aorta, which ordinarily leads to a progressive increase in vessel wall stiffness [13]. These effects of perindopril and indapamide were demonstrated in a clinical trial where control was associated with baseline pulse wave velocity and the use of these two drugs [14].

ORTHOSTATIC HYPOTENSION: A COMPLICATION, A RISK

Asymptomatic orthostatic hypotension (OH) is defined as a drop in SBP of 20 mmHg or a drop in DBP of 10 mmHg from supine to standing after three 3 minutes [15]. Symptomatic OH is defined as dizziness, lightheadedness, or fainting when a patient goes from the supine to standing position. The causes of OH can be cardiogenic, neurocardiogenic or neurogenic. Orthostatic hypotension is more common among the older population, with prevalence rates as high as 18–33%. Orthostatic hypotension is one of the leading causes of falls in the elderly. For example, in one study of nursing home patients with a history of a fall, OH was the most probable cause in 15% and a contributing cause in 26% of the patients [16, 17]. Orthostatic hypotension is more commonly seen in patients with either a high PP form of hypertension or isolated systolic hypertension (ISH). It is not clear whether OH and ISH are merely a consequence of old age or if ISH is directly related to OH. Some antihypertensive medications, like α-blockers, β-blockers, nitrates, vasodilators and calcium channel blockers, can cause OH. Particular medications, like α-blockers, have a first dose effect that is exaggerated if the patient is volume-contracted; however, patients accommodate to these drugs and often the occurrence of OH decreases with continued usage. More conservative antihypertensive treatment, starting with lower doses of drugs with careful upward titration in patients with OH, is recommended as a safety precaution. In our experience, low dose clonidine at night-time, when the BP is the highest due to the supine position, appears to control the BP at night and also decrease the incidence of OH during the day time.

HYPERTENSION IN KIDNEY DISEASE

Hypertension is the second most common cause of ESRD. Hypertension is both a cause and result of CKD, and affects both normal and damaged kidneys. The kidneys have a very sophisticated hemodynamic autoregulatory mechanism that maintains steady renal perfusion between mean arterial pressures ranging from 80 to 160 mmHg. This autoregulatory capacity is reduced both in long-term hypertension and by accelerated hypertension if even present for a short period of time. In chronic hypertension, there is an increase in glomerular capillary hydrostatic pressure, which is one factor that leads to the development of glomerulosclerosis in the patient with hypertension. Accelerated hypertension speeds this process up, often leading to acute kidney injury (AKI) and, if not adequately treated, progressing to advanced CKD, if not ESRD.

Both the JNC-7 and the National Kidney Foundation (NKF) Kidney Disease Outcome Quality Initiative (KDOQI) guidelines [18] recommend that BP values be maintained below 130/80 mmHg for all patients diagnosed with CKD in order to slow the progression of kidney damage and also to reduce CV complications. The Modification of Diet in Renal Disease (MDRD) study [18] demonstrated the adverse effects of hypertension on the kidneys. In this study, the decline in glomerular filtration rate (GFR) was significantly slower in the low BP group (MAP goal ≤92 mmHg) than in the usual BP group (MAP goal ≤107 mmHg). The lower blood pressure group had fewer patients with a rapid loss of GFR progressing to ESRD compared to the usual blood pressure group. There was no significant difference in the rate of complications with treatment between these two groups. A subgroup of the Systolic Hypertension in the Elderly Program (SHEP) evaluated the effects of systolic, diastolic, mean arterial and PP on rate of change of GFR. Higher SBPs were more strongly related to the decline in GFR when compared to diastolic pressures. The relative risk for worsening of kidney function for a SBP elevation of 9 mmHg was 1.38, compared to 1.06 for an 8 mmHg elevation in DBP. This study demonstrated that treating isolated systolic hypertension in the elderly can slow functional decline.

Proteinuria, together with hypertension, plays a significant role in loss of renal function and increases the risk of CV diseases in both diabetic and non-diabetic patients. Proteinuria acts as a surrogate for kidney injury even before the development of overt manifestations of kidney damage. Baseline proteinuria is a very important predictor of GFR decline. There is a noteworthy increase in CV disease risk in the patient with hypertension and proteinuria. The BP goal for patients with proteinuria as recommended by the American Diabetes Association and the National Kidney Foundation is <130/80 mmHg. Once this BP goal has been reached the emphasis is shifted to control of proteinuria (spot urine protein/creatinine ratio <200 mg/g) with the optimal use of antiproteinuric antihypertensive medications, such as those that block the renin-angiotensin system (RAS).

ANTIHYPERTENSIVES IN KIDNEY DISEASE

Renin-angiotensin system inhibitors are the antihypertensive drugs of choice in patients with CKD. Angiotensin converting enzyme (ACE) inhibitors and angiotensin receptor blockers (ARBs) are considered the first line of treatment in these patients. In the African-American Study of Kidney Diseases (AASK) the ACE inhibitor ramipril was compared to the calcium channel blocker (CCB) amlodipine or the β-blocker metoprolol in African-American patients with hypertensive glomerulosclerosis. Treatment with ramipril showed a greater benefit in slowing the deterioration of renal function, a greater decrease in proteinuria, a decreased incidence of ESRD and deaths from all causes [20]. Similarly, ARBs have significant renoprotective effects which are independent of the level to which they reduce BP [21].

The major side-effects of the ACE inhibitor drug class are a reversible form of worsening renal function, hyperkalemia, cough and angioedema. In patients with hypertension and CKD, it is not unusual to see a slight rise in creatinine (fall in GFR) as the BP improves and/or there is exposure to either an ACE inhibitor or an ARB. Impairment of renal autoregulation from long standing hypertension can explain this increase in creatinine as there is a drop in afferent arterial pressure when systemic BP is brought down. Apperloo and co-workers assessed renal function in patients with mild-to-moderate renal insufficiency after they had received an ACE inhibitor [22]. During the next four-years of follow-up, the initial fall in renal function remained stable in patients with moderate renal insufficiency and renal function recovered nearly completely after ACE inhibitor therapy was stopped [23]. The reversibility of renal function indicated that the initial changes were due to hemodynamic changes (reduction in intraglomerular pressures) and not structural changes.

When there is an initial increase in creatinine (greater than 30%) or repeated measurements show a progressive increase, the appropriate response to ACE inhibitor therapy is to discontinue the compound in question and to look for other causes of renal failure if function does not return to its original baseline. The decline in GFR may be less severe with ARBs compared to ACE inhibitors. Angiotensin-receptor blockers block angiotensin II type I (AT_1) receptors causing efferent vasodilation but also stimulate angiotensin II type II (AT_2) receptors causing afferent vasodilation, thereby maintaining the GFR. This is, however, hypothetical and there is currently no clinical trial evidence favoring one of these drug classes over the other based on their capacity to reduce renal function.

Hyperkalemia is another complication that can occur in patients with renal insufficiency when treated with either an ACE inhibitor or an ARB. Discontinuing any drugs that can independently increase the potassium level such as non-steroidal anti-inflammatory drugs (NSAIDs) or salt substitutes, prescribing low doses of either an ACE inhibitor or an ARB, and/or using loop or thiazide diuretics can minimize this complication. There is preliminary evidence that proteinuria reduction may be more substantial with a combination of ARB and ACE inhibitors or high-dose RAS inhibition; however, there is an ongoing study to evaluate the capacity of combined ACE inhibitor and ARB therapy to afford better renoprotection than either therapy alone [24, 25]. A new class of drugs, direct renin inhibitors (e.g. aliskiren), is currently being studied. When used in combination with ACE inhibitors or ARBs they have been shown to significantly improve proteinuria with very small additional changes in BP; they are therefore considered safe in patients with proteinuria and well-controlled BP [26].

Calcium channel blockers, like verapamil and diltiazem, and β-blockers, have also been demonstrated to have some antiproteinuric effects, although less than what is seen with RAS inhibitors. These drugs can be used as add on drugs when the patient has significant proteinuria or poorly controlled hypertension in a patient already taking, or intolerant to, either an ACE inhibitor or an ARB.

HYPERTENSION IN DIABETES

Diabetes mellitus is the most common cause of ESRD, adult blindness and amputation, and is a major risk factor for CV and cerebrovascular complications. Compared to a 25% prevalence of hypertension in the general adult population, hypertension is present in 75% of diabetic patients. Both diabetes and hypertension are independent risk factors for cardiac, renal and vascular damage. A combination of these two conditions increases both the microvascular and macrovascular complications substantially. Multiple studies have demonstrated the benefits of lowering BP in diabetics. In order to reduce the morbidity of diabetes mellitus, BP should be maintained <130/80 mmHg in these patients.

The United Kingdom Prospective Diabetes Study (UKPDS) was a multicenter trial evaluating the difference in incidence of multiple diabetes related endpoints (sudden death, death from hyperglycemia, fatal or non-fatal myocardial infarction, renal failure, amputation, vitreous hemorrhage, retinal photocoagulation, blindness and cataract extraction) and death in two different BP treatment groups [27]. A cohort of 1148 patients with hypertension and diabetes were divided into tight BP control (<150/85 mmHg) and less tight BP control (180/105 mmHg) groups. After 10 years of follow-up, there was a significant difference in risk for major health events in these two BP groups. The tight BP group had a relative risk reduction of 24% for diabetes related endpoints, 32% for diabetes related deaths, 44% for strokes and 37% for microvascular diseases. Schrier and colleagues studied the benefits on diabetes related endpoints (decline in renal function, development of retinopathy, nephropathy and CV diseases) of treating normotensive (mean DBP between 80 and 89 mmHg) diabetic patients. Patients were randomly assigned to one of two treatment strategies: intensive treatment with the goal of decreasing the DBP by 10 mmHg from the mean baseline value (target DBP < 75 mmHg) (with further random assignment to receive either nisoldipine or enalapril), or moderate treatment with no intended change in the baseline DBP (these patients were thus randomly assigned to receive placebo) [28]. The achieved BP in the intensive treatment and moderate treatment BP groups was 132/78 and 138/86 mmHg, respectively. There was no significant difference in creatinine clearance between both treatment groups during the 5-year follow-up period. With intensive BP treatment there was also no difference between the interventions with regard to individuals progressing from normoalbuminuria to microalbuminuria (25% intensive therapy vs. 18% moderate therapy, $P = 0.20$) or microalbuminuria to overt albuminuria (16% intensive therapy vs. 23% moderate therapy, $P = 0.28$). Over the 5-year follow-up period, there was no difference between the intensive and moderate groups with regard to the progression of diabetic retinopathy and neuropathy. Intensive therapy did, however, demonstrate a lower overall incidence of deaths, 5.5% vs. 10.7%, $P = 0.037$.

ANTIHYPERTENSIVES IN DIABETES

Hypertension and diabetes usually present as a part of the metabolic syndrome, along with obesity and dyslipidemia. Control of hypertension reduces renal, microvascular and macrovascular complications in both diabetic and metabolic syndrome patients, but different antihypertensive medication classes have variable beneficial effects. Most commonly, multidrug therapy is necessary to effectively treat hypertension in the diabetic population. The RAS blockers have become the standard of care in the last two decades for hypertensive diabetics for both their cardiac and renal protection. ACE inhibitors and ARBs have significant effects on decreasing morbidity and complications associated with diabetes mellitus seemingly in a BP-independent manner. In addition, they are associated with a reduced risk of new onset diabetes in patients with impaired glucose tolerance.

In the MICRO Heart Outcomes Protection Evaluation (HOPE) study, the benefits of the ACE inhibitor ramipril over placebo were striking. Patients in the ramipril group had a significant risk reduction of myocardial infarction, stroke, and all cause cardiac mortality [29]. Similarly, ramipril was shown to slow the progression of renal damage, and risk of developing ESRD. Ramipril showed a beneficial effect on proteinuria by both decreasing the incidence of new proteinuria in normal patients and also by decreasing the amount of protein in already proteinuric patients. Similar results were found with the ARB, losartan, on CV and renal protection in the Reduction of Endpoints in NIDDM with the Angiotensin II Antagonist Losartan (RENAAL) study [30]. Thiazides have also shown to decrease CV risk in patients with diabetes, but these drugs in high doses should be used with caution as they can worsen glucose intolerance.

A recently completed trial demonstrates the effectiveness and safety of aggressively lowering BP in patients with diabetes [31]. Howard and colleagues randomized patients with type 2 diabetes to reach more aggressive BP and low density lipoprotein (LDL) levels than previously studied. The patients were 499 American Indian men and women aged 40 years or older who were brought to an LDL-C of 70 mg/dl or lower, and a SBP of 115 mmHg or lower versus a LDL-C value less than 100 mg/dl and a SBP less than 130 mmHg. Although clinical events were no different between the groups, carotid intima-media thickness regressed in the aggressive group and progressed in the standard group (–0.012 mm vs. 0.038 mm; P <0.001). Left ventricular mass index also was reduced (–2.4 g/m (2.7) vs. –1.2 g/m (2.7); P = 0.03) more in the aggressive therapy group.

BLOOD PRESSURE AND CARDIOVASCULAR DISEASE

Cardiovascular disease is the number one cause of mortality in adult and elderly populations in the United States and many other developed and developing nations. Medical care for coronary artery disease (CAD) puts a heavy demand on medical resources throughout the world. Hypertension is considered a very important modifiable risk factor in these conditions. Importantly, 75% of hypertensive patients have other risk factors for CVD, such as hyperlipidemia, DM, and obesity. Hypertension has an additive effect on the risk for CVD when present with these other conditions. Several studies have demonstrated that systolic and diastolic BPs have a strong association with CAD. A graded increase in CAD related mortality and morbidity is seen with progressive increases in BP.

Though it is proven beyond doubt that hypertension has a positive association with CAD, the question commonly asked is *"what is the optimal BP to decrease this risk?"*. In an observational analysis by Vasan and co-workers, a large population of 6859 patients from the Framingham study was followed for a mean of 11.1 years to study the impact of BP pressure on the incidence of CV diseases. The study population was divided into three groups: optimal BP (<120/80 mmHg), normal BP (SBP 120–129, DBP 80–84 mmHg), and high normal BP (SBP 130–139, DBP 85–89 mmHg). The primary outcome was the time to occurrence of any of the following major CV events: death due to CVD, myocardial infarction, stroke or HF. The CV event rates increased in a stepwise manner across the different BP ranges. Among younger subjects (35–64 years) there was an observed difference in the incidence of CVD in the high normal group with a higher incidence among men. In the older population, there was no such sex dependent difference in the incidence of CVD. Importantly, in both age groups and sexes, there was a significant increase for CV events in patients with normal and high normal blood pressure compared to those with optimal BP (Figure 5.3) [32].

ANTIHYPERTENSIVES IN CARDIAC CONDITIONS

All patients with uncontrolled hypertension are considered to be at risk of developing HF. For this reason, all patients with hypertension are now classified as Stage A HF by the American College of Cardiology and the American Heart Association (ACC/AHA). It is critical to tightly control BP in patients with HF to prevent further damage to the myocardium and to decrease mortality. Different drug classes have been shown to decrease

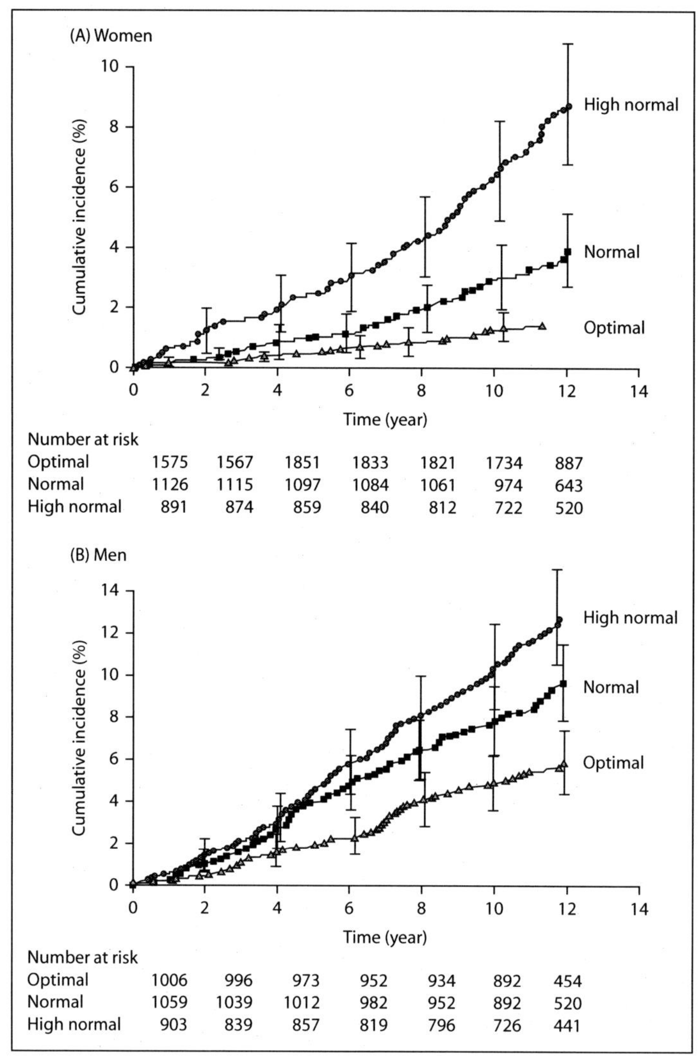

Figure 5.3 Cumulative incidence of cardiovascular events in women (Panel A) and men (Panel B) without hypertension, according to blood-pressure category at the baseline examination.

HF-related symptoms as well as the mortality, which attends this disease. ACE inhibitors have been shown to decrease the risk of developing HF and myocardial infarction when given to patients with asymptomatic left ventricular failure as well as in patients with all classes of HF [33]. Angiotensin receptor blockers are as effective, or slightly less effective, in risk reduction compared to ACE inhibitors and are considered as second line treatment to be used when patients are intolerant of ACE inhibitors [34].

Along with ACE inhibitors, β-blockers are considered mainstay therapies in the treatment of HF. Beta-blockers, like metoprolol, carvedilol, and bisoprolol, are recommended in all patients with systolic forms of HF, unless contravening conditions exist. Metoprolol has shown to prolong survival, reduce the need for hospitalization, and improve New York Heart Association (NYHA) functional class [35]. Aldosterone receptor antagonists also improve survival in patients with HF but have not demonstrated any benefits in patients with asymptomatic left ventricular failure [36]. These drugs should be used with caution as they can cause severe hyperkalemia when used in combination with ACE inhibitors. Nitrates, thiazide and loop diuretics improve symptoms in patients with HF but do not appear to have any significant effect in reducing mortality. Myocardial infarction is the leading cause of HF in the United States and BP can be quite variable largely dependent on proximity to the event. Therapeutic measures should be aimed at:

1. Increasing coronary artery patency and reducing the initial infarct size with the early use of aspirin and reperfusion therapy; and
2. Preventing or slowing remodeling and the late loss of myocardial function with RAS inhibitors and possibly β-blockers.

Blood pressure control in these patients should typically incorporate both an ACE inhibitor and a β-blocker. Oftentimes, diuretic and/or CCB therapy is required with these therapies if BP is to be effectively reduced. The inclusion of both an ACE inhibitor and a β-blocker in the treatment regimen following a myocardial infarction has a clinical trial basis in that long term use of ACE inhibitors following a myocardial infarction have been shown to delay the onset of HF in patients with asymptomatic left ventricular failure as well as to prolong survival. Beta-blockers, when started post myocardial infarction, also improve survival and reduce the rate of both sudden death and recurrent myocardial infarction independent of left ventricular function.

SUMMARY

The optimal targets for systolic and diastolic BP remain unknown, but we now have growing evidence that lower BP in patients with diabetes, renal disease and HF are well tolerated. Moreover, the DBP in isolated systolic hypertension and wide PP hypertension does not appear to be substantially affected with active treatment of the hypertension. Despite everything we know about the benefits and safety of treating hypertension, control rates remain poor. Physicians are hesitant to titrate currently available medications for fear of dangers associated with aggressive treatment or they may simply not know how to titrate the drugs.

Patients with poorly controlled BP are at increased risk of developing CV and cerebrovascular morbidity and mortality and therefore may represent a substantial burden to healthcare resources. Identifying the optimal BP levels in patients with various morbidities and treating BP more aggressively, perhaps with multiple drugs, can significantly lower the risks of these disease. Ongoing trials to define these optimal BP levels are urgently needed.

ACKNOWLEDGMENTS

We would like to thank Tia A. Paul, University of Maryland School of Medicine, Baltimore, MD, for expert secretarial assistance.

REFERENCES

1. Burt VL, Whelton P, Roccella EJ *et al*. Prevalence of hypertension in the US adult population. Results from the Third National Health and Nutrition Examination Survey, 1988–1991. *Hypertension* 1995; 25:305–313.
2. World Health Organization. World Health Report 2002: Reducing Risks, Promoting Healthy Life. Campanini, B. 1–248. 2002. Geneva, Switzerland. Ref Type: Report.
3. Chobanian AV, Bakris GL, Black HR *et al*. The seventh report of the Joint National Committee on Prevention, Detection, Evaluation, and Treatment of High Blood Pressure. *JAMA* 2003; 289:2560–2572.

4. Franklin SS, Sutton-Tyrrell K, Belle SH, Weber MA, Kuller LH. The importance of pulsatile components of hypertension in predicting carotid stenosis in older adults. *J Hypertens* 1997; 15:1143–1150.

5. Franklin SS. Cardiovascular risks related to increased diastolic, systolic and pulse pressure. An epidemiologist's point of view. *Pathol Biol (Paris)* 1999; 47:594–603.

6. Domanski M, Mitchell G, Pfeffer M *et al*. Pulse pressure and cardiovascular disease-related mortality: follow-up study of the Multiple Risk Factor Intervention Trial (MRFIT). *JAMA* 2002; 287:2677–2683.

7. Pastor-Barriuso R, Banegas JR, Damian J, Appel LJ, Guallar E. Systolic blood pressure, diastolic blood pressure, and pulse pressure: an evaluation of their joint effect on mortality. *Ann Intern Med* 2003; 139:731–739.

8. Hansson L, Zanchetti A, Carruthers SG *et al*. Effects of intensive blood-pressure lowering and low-dose aspirin in patients with hypertension: principal results of the Hypertension Optimal Treatment (HOT) randomised trial. HOT Study Group. *Lancet* 1998; 351:1755–1762.

9. Stewart IM. Relation of reduction in pressure to first myocardial infarction in patients receiving treatment for severe hypertension. *Lancet* 1979; 1:861–865.

10. Cruickshank JM, Thorp JM, Zacharias FJ. Benefits and potential harm of lowering high blood pressure. *Lancet* 1987; 1:581–584.

11. Cushman WC, Materson BJ, Williams DW, Reda DJ. Pulse pressure changes with six classes of antihypertensive agents in a randomized, controlled trial. *Hypertension* 2001; 38:953–957.

12. Materson BJ, Reda DJ, Cushman WC *et al*. Single-drug therapy for hypertension in men. A comparison of six antihypertensive agents with placebo. The Department of Veterans Affairs Cooperative Study Group on Antihypertensive Agents. *N Engl J Med* 1993; 328:914–921.

13. Levy BI, Curmi P, Poitevin P, Safar ME. Modifications of the arterial mechanical properties of normotensive and hypertensive rats without arterial pressure changes. *J Cardiovasc Pharmacol* 1989; 14:253–259.

14. Protogerou A, Blacher J, Stergiou GS, Achimastos A, Safar ME. Blood pressure response under chronic antihypertensive drug therapy: the role of aortic stiffness in the REASON (Preterax in Regression of Arterial Stiffness in a Controlled Double-Blind) Study. *J Am Coll Cardiol* 2009; 53:445–451.

15. Beckett NS, Peters R, Fletcher AE *et al*. Treatment of hypertension in patients 80 years of age or older. *N Engl J Med* 2008; 358:1887–1898.

16. Lipsitz LA. Orthostatic hypotension in the elderly. *N Engl J Med* 1989; 321:952–957.

17. Rutan GH, Hermanson B, Bild DE, Kittner SJ, LaBaw F, Tell GS. Orthostatic hypotension in older adults. The Cardiovascular Health Study. CHS Collaborative Research Group. *Hypertension* 1992; 19:508–519.

18. Hunsicker LG, Adler S, Caggiula A *et al*. Predictors of the progression of renal disease in the Modification of Diet in Renal Disease Study. *Kidney Int* 1997; 51:1908–1919.

19. KDOQI clinical practice guidelines for management of dyslipidemias in patients with kidney disease: evaluation, classification, and stratification. *Am J Kidney Dis* 2003; I–IV, S1–S91.

20. Agodoa LY, Appel L, Bakris GL *et al*. Effect of ramipril vs amlodipine on renal outcomes in hypertensive nephrosclerosis: a randomized controlled trial. *JAMA* 2001; 285:2719–2728.

21. Lewis EJ, Hunsicker LG, Clarke WR *et al*. Renoprotective effect of the angiotensin-receptor antagonist irbesartan in patients with nephropathy due to type 2 diabetes. *N Engl J Med* 2001; 345:851–860.

22. Apperloo AJ, de Zeeuw D, de Jong PE. Discordant effects of enalapril and lisinopril on systemic and renal hemodynamics. *Clin Pharmacol Ther* 1994; 56:647–658.

23. Palmer BF. Renal dysfunction complicating the treatment of hypertension. *N Engl J Med* 2002; 347:1256–1261.

24. The ONTARGET Investigators. Telmisartan, ramipril, or both in patients at high risk for vascular events. *N Engl J Med* 2008;NEJMoa0801317.

25. Vogt L, Laverman GD, de Zeeuw D, Navis G. The COOPERATE trial. *Lancet* 2003; 361:1055–1056.

26. Estacio RO, Jeffers BW, Gifford N, Schrier RW. Effect of blood pressure control on diabetic microvascular complications in patients with hypertension and type 2 diabetes. *Diabetes Care* 2000; 23:B54–B64.

27. Holman RR, Paul SK, Bethel MA, Matthews DR, Neil HA. 10-year follow-up of intensive glucose control in type 2 diabetes. *N Engl J Med* 2008; 359:1577–1589.

28. Schrier RW, Estacio RO, Jeffers B. Appropriate blood pressure control in NIDDM (ABCD) Trial. *Diabetologia* 1996; 39:1646–1654.

29. Jones SC, Bowes PD, Hall E, Connolly V, Kelly WF, Bilous RW. HOPE for patients with type 2 diabetes: an application of the findings of the MICRO-HOPE substudy in a British hospital diabetes clinic. *Diabet Med* 2001; 18:667–670.

30. Brenner BM, Cooper ME, de Zeeuw D *et al*. Effects of losartan on renal and cardiovascular outcomes in patients with type 2 diabetes and nephropathy. *N Engl J Med* 2001; 345:861–869.

31. Howard BV, Roman MJ, Devereux RB *et al*. Effect of lower targets for blood pressure and LDL cholesterol on atherosclerosis in diabetes: the SANDS randomized trial. *JAMA* 2008; 299:1678–1689.

32. Vasan RS, Larson MG, Leip EP *et al*. Impact of high-normal blood pressure on the risk of cardiovascular disease. *N Engl J Med* 2001; 345:1291–1297.

33. Garg R, Yusuf S. Overview of randomized trials of angiotensin-converting enzyme inhibitors on mortality and morbidity in patients with heart failure. Collaborative Group on ACE Inhibitor Trials. *JAMA* 1995; 273:1450–1456.

34. Jessup M, Abraham WT, Casey DE *et al*. 2009 Focused Update: ACCF/AHA Guidelines for the Diagnosis and Management of Heart Failure in Adults: A Report of the American College of Cardiology Foundation/American Heart Association Task Force on Practice Guidelines: Developed in Collaboration With the International Society for Heart and Lung Transplantation. *Circulation* 2009; 119:1977–2016.

35. Hjalmarson A, Goldstein S, Fagerberg B *et al*. Effects of controlled-release metoprolol on total mortality, hospitalizations, and well-being in patients with heart failure: the Metoprolol CR/XL Randomized Intervention Trial in congestive Heart Failure (MERIT-HF). MERIT-HF Study Group. *JAMA* 2000; 283:1295–1302.

36. Pitt B. Aldosterone blockade in patients with heart failure and a reduced left ventricular ejection fraction. *Eur Heart J* 2009; 30:387–388.

6

Exercise, athletes and blood pressure

J. J. Leddy, J. L. Izzo Jr.

BACKGROUND

Because of their apparently high level of fitness, athletes and physically active persons are often thought to be free of cardiovascular disease and hypertension (HTN). While the prevalence of HTN in these groups is approximately 50% that of the general population [1], and while exercise is an important non-pharmacologic intervention for the prevention [2] and treatment [3] of elevated blood pressure (BP), some athletes and physically active patients are at greater risk for being hypertensive. These include African Americans, the elderly, the obese, and athletes with diabetes mellitus, renal disease, or a family history of hypertension. Elevated BP is one of the most common abnormalities found during the sports pre-participation physical evaluation (PPE) [4] of athletes and HTN remains the most common cardiovascular condition encountered in athletic populations [5], so all athletes require screening for HTN.

This chapter will:
1. Acquaint clinicians with the evidence for the effects of exercise on BP and on HTN incidence;
2. Review the BP patterns seen in athletes and the physically active;
3. Discuss the risk factors and the important history elements and physical examination procedures used in the clinical evaluation of HTN in athletes;
4. Review the treatment options for the hypertensive athlete; and
5. Give clinicians information to allow them to make specific sports participation recommendations for athletes with HTN.

The goals are to present the issues that the hypertensive athlete raises for practitioners and to give practitioners information that helps them to evaluate and manage elevated BP readings in athletes. Questions to be addressed that will highlight these issues include:

1. What are the most important elements in taking a history in the athlete with HTN?
2. What is the best type of exercise for a particular patient/athlete?
3. What lifestyle modifications are most germane to the athlete with HTN?

John J. Leddy, MD, FACSM, FACP, Associate Professor of Clinical Orthopaedics, Assistant Professor of Medicine, Family Medicine, Rehabilitation Sciences and Nutrition, Research Assistant Professor of Physiology, University Sports Medicine, State University of New York at Buffalo, School.

Joseph L. Izzo Jr., MD, FACP, FAHA, Professor of Medicine, Professor of Pharmacology and Toxicology, Clinical Director of Medicine, State University of New York at Buffalo, School of Medicine and Biomedical Sciences and the Erie County Medical Center, Buffalo, NY, USA.

4. What are the best medications for the treatment of HTN in the athlete from an efficacy and side-effect point of view?

EXERCISE TRAINING AND BLOOD PRESSURE

Athletes are engaged in various forms of regular physical activity and physical training to improve fitness and athletic performance. Physical activity is defined as voluntary movements produced by skeletal muscles that result in energy expenditure [6], while aerobic exercise is defined as rhythmic exercise of large muscle groups (e.g., running, walking, cycling, swimming, rowing, etc.) that increases respiratory and heart rates and oxygen consumption [7]. Cardiorespiratory fitness is a physiological attribute related to the efficiency of supply of oxygen to the muscles during sustained physical activity that is increased by progressive aerobic exercise training [6]. Aerobic exercise tends to increase cardiac preload while resistance exercise, particularly power lifting, tends to increase left ventricular afterload [7].

Epidemiological studies have shown that both physical activity [8] and cardiorespiratory fitness [2] are inversely related to BP levels and HTN incidence, while randomized clinical trials have proved that physical activity is effective at reducing BP in normotensive, pre-hypertensive and hypertensive persons [3]. In the aggregate, studies confirm that aerobic exercise training reduces mean systolic BP by 2–7 mmHg, with the greatest reduction in hypertensive patients [3]. Most trials have employed exercise regimens that used a frequency (on most, preferably all, days of the week), intensity (moderate, i.e. 40–60% of peak oxygen consumption, which can be estimated clinically by taking 40–60% of age predicted maximum heart rate according to the formula 220 minus age in years), and duration (≥30 min of continuous or accumulated physical activity per day) based on the American College of Sports Medicine (ACSM) prescription for improving cardiorespiratory fitness [7]. Some studies suggest that cardiorespiratory fitness has a more powerful antihypertensive effect than physical activity [9, 10] in a dose–response relationship [10] but this has not been universally observed [11, 12]. Individual preference is an important factor to maximize long-term adherence to exercise [7] and studies show that persons will be more successful at this if the intensity is moderate [13]. Moderate intensity exercise corresponds to a rating of perceived exertion (RPE) of 4–6 (on a scale of 0–10) where the breathing rate is increased but the person is capable of carrying on a conversation [14]. The ACSM recommends primarily endurance physical activity that can also be supplemented by resistance exercise [7]. Moderate intensity resistance training that emphasizes lower weight, higher repetition regimens has been observed to lower mean systolic BP from 3–6 mmHg [15].

The mechanisms for the effect of exercise training on BP are thought primarily to reflect neurochemical and structural changes that reduce peripheral vascular resistance (PVR) [7]. Exercise training lowers PVR via a number of avenues:

1. Reduced norepinephrine release.
2. Reduced insulin-induced sympathetic nervous stimulation.
3. Reduced release and activity of the potent local vasoconstrictor endothelin-1.
4. Increased release of the potent local vasodilator nitric oxide.
5. Vascular remodeling (i.e. increased cross sectional capillary density and increased arterial luminal diameter and greater arterial compliance) [7].

BLOOD PRESSURE PATTERNS IN ATHLETES AND PHYSICALLY ACTIVE PEOPLE

SUSTAINED HYPERTENSION

While the overall prevalence of HTN in the physically active is approximately 50% lower than in the general population [1], athletes who are African American, elderly, obese, diabetic or who have chronic kidney disease have a higher risk of developing HTN. Almost 80% of adolescents found to have a BP above 142/92 mmHg during a PPE eventually develop chronically elevated BP [4]; therefore, BP should be closely monitored in all physically active individuals. Most athletes with HTN have essential HTN and the prevalence of secondary causes of HTN is the same as in the general population [16]. Wheelchair athletes with spinal cord injuries may also have severe episodic HTN related to autonomic dysfunction [17].

WHITE COAT HYPERTENSION

Out-of-office BP recordings (home BP in the morning and evening or 24-h ambulatory BP monitoring, ABPM) should be obtained in anyone with elevated office readings. It is critical to avoid a cavalier diagnosis of HTN because athletes often have the 'white coat effect' (marked home–office BP difference). In a study of 410 athletes (aged 16.4±2.6 years) [18], 18 hypertensives (4.4%) were detected and evaluated with 24-hr ABPM. Sixteen of these had "white coat hypertension" (normal 24-h average, daytime and nocturnal BP). In "white coat HTN", the risk profile for cardiovascular disease is much closer to that of normotension than to sustained HTN, thus athletes with 'white coat HTN' usually do not require drug therapy. In this group, BP should be monitored at least yearly and appropriate steps taken if the BP elevation becomes sustained.

ISOLATED SYSTOLIC HYPERTENSION

Many conditioned athletes (particularly young men) have "athlete's heart" with very high resting stroke volume and cardiac output with low PVR and heart rate [19]. Pulse pressure and systolic BP are high in these individuals because cardiac stroke volume is so high, very often in the range of pre-hypertension and occasionally in the range of stage 1 HTN [20, 21]. Diastolic BP is usually normal.

SPURIOUS SYSTOLIC HYPERTENSION

Another anomaly of systolic BP in athletes is "spurious systolic hypertension" or SSH, which is believed to be the result of exaggerated pulse pressure amplification in the arm as detected by arterial tonometry. In affected individuals, central (aortic) BP may be substantially less (30–40 mmHg) than arm BP. What is not known at present is the long-term significance of this condition. Using a definition for SSH as a brachial systolic BP >140 with a central systolic BP <124 mmHg for males and <120 mmHg for females, Hulsen and colleagues [22] found 57 cases in young men and only three cases in young women among the 750 participants in the Atherosclerosis Risk in Young Adults study. Twenty-year Framingham risk scores in the SSH group based on brachial diastolic BP values were not significantly different from those of normotensives.

EVALUATION OF HYPERTENSION IN ATHLETES

What are the most important elements in taking a history in the athlete with hypertension?
The athlete should be questioned about family history of HTN and premature cardiovascular disease as well as behavioral factors including high intake of sodium and saturated fats (especially in processed and 'fast' foods), alcohol, drugs (specifically, stimulants and cocaine), tobacco, human growth hormone or anabolic steroids (Table 6.1). Alcohol consumption is not uncommon in scholastic athletes [23], the use of which in the evening can raise BP readings in the morning and abstinence may be therapeutic. Athletes may be taking other substances that increase BP, including non-steroidal anti-inflammatory drugs (NSAIDs), caffeine, diet pills, decongestants, herbal and dietary supplements, which often contain "natural"

Table 6.1 Athlete behaviors and medications that can increase blood pressure.

Sodium and saturated fat intake (fast foods)
Alcohol
Tobacco (any form)
OTC meds
– Cold remedies, decongestants
– "Diet pills" containing phenylpropanolamine (banned since 2005)
Ergogenic Aides
– Caffeine
– Pseudoephedrine (Sudafed®)
– Cocaine
– Human Growth Hormone
– Anabolic Steroids
Prescription Medications
– NSAIDs*
– Oral Contraceptives
Dietary Supplements
– Guanara
– Ephedra (banned since 2004)
– Ma huang
*Also available over-the-counter

stimulants such as guarana, ma huang, or ephedra. Females should be questioned about oral contraceptive use since about 5% develop HTN over a 5-year period [24]. Symptoms related to BP elevation should also be identified, including any exertional chest pain, unusual dyspnea, or declining athletic performance.

PHYSICAL EXAMINATION

At least two pressures should be recorded for each visit. BP determinations should be made according to standardized guidelines: undisturbed in a quiet room after at least 5 minutes, back supported in a chair, feet on the floor, arm supported at the level of the heart, and without talking. It is especially critical to use a properly sized cuff where the bladder encircles at least 80% of arm circumference to avoid misleadingly high readings [24]; an obese adult size cuff for a mid-arm circumference >33 cm and a child's cuff for mid-arm circumference <23 cm should be used [25, 26]. The cuff must be inflated to at least 20 mm greater than the inflation values associated with disappearance of the radial pulse to avoid the "auscultatory gap" and so potentially underestimate BP [25, 26]. Blood pressure readings should be taken in both arms; if the pressures differ, the arm with the higher pressure should be used. If the initial values are elevated, two other sets of readings should be obtained at least 1 week apart [27].

If the arm pressure is elevated, a measurement in one leg (particularly in patients less than 30 years old) is indicated. To measure leg BP, an appropriately sized cuff should be applied to the mid-thigh with the individual lying supine with auscultation over the popliteal artery [28]. Leg systolic BP is usually 10–20% greater than the brachial systolic BP due to peripheral BP amplification [29]. If the leg systolic BP is less than the brachial systolic BP, peripheral arterial disease should be considered in older patients and coarctation of the aorta in younger patients. If an elevated BP is found, a careful funduscopic examination, thyroid gland palpation, cardiac auscultation, abdominal auscultation (for a renal bruit), and simultaneous palpation of the radial and femoral pulses (a delay should prompt evaluation for coarctation of the aorta) should be undertaken.

In adolescents, BP varies by age, sex, and height [30] according to easily accessible tables (www.nhlbi.nih.gov/guidelines/hypertension/child_tbl.htm). Normal BP is defined as <90th percentile; high normal is 90–95th percentile; HTN is >95–99th percentile; and severe HTN is >99th percentile for age, sex and height, respectively. These categories correspond to the adult categories of normal (BP <120/80 mmHg), pre-hypertension (systolic BP 120–139 mmHg or diastolic BP 80–89 mmHg), stage 1 (systolic BP 140–159 mmHg or diastolic BP 90–99 mmHg) and stage 2 (systolic BP ≥160 mmHg or diastolic BP ≥100 mmHg) HTN.

TARGET ORGAN ASSESSMENT

Once a diagnosis of HTN has been established, athletes (adults and children) should undergo evaluation to assess the pattern of end-organ damage and, in selected cases, identifiable causes of HTN. Secondary HTN develops in fewer than 5% of athletes [16]. It tends to be present in younger patients, adult patients with rapid onset of severe HTN, and patients with HTN that responds poorly to routine therapies. The true prevalence rates of secondary HTN are not known. In young women, the most common secondary cause of hypertension is fibromuscular hyperplasia of one or both renal arteries [31]. Other less common causes include increased adrenal steroid or catecholamine production, coarctation of the aorta, and hyperthyroidism. Athletes with pre-hypertension (90–95th percentile in adolescents) and stage 1 HTN (95–99th percentile in adolescents) should have blood chemistries and a lipid profile, hematocrit, urinalysis, and an electrocardiogram. Athletes with stage 2 HTN (>99th percentile in adolescents), abnormal lab results, or a possible secondary cause of HTN should be referred for additional study, including echocardiography and therapy [5, 27, 30].

It is recommended that any athlete with sustained HTN have echocardiography [27, 30]. The interpretation of increased myocardial mass in athletes can be difficult. In general, athletes develop a pattern of physiologic "eccentric hypertrophy" in which increased left ventricular (LV) mass is associated with normal or increased fractional mid-wall shortening, high LV volume, and normal or minimally increased LV wall thickness. At the extremes, this pattern is easily differentiated from the pathologic "concentric hypertrophy" of hypertension, where the LV chamber size is normal or reduced and the LV wall thickness is increased [32]. Concentric hypertrophy is also found in bodybuilders. Hypertensive athletes with ambiguous findings on echocardiography require cardiology consultation. Left ventricular hypertrophy beyond the "athlete's heart" should limit participation until the BP is normalized [27, 30], which may be a problem for a few highly trained athletes. The possibility of hypertrophic cardiomyopathy should always be considered under these circumstances [5, 19].

PARTICIPATION RECOMMENDATIONS FOR ATHLETES WITH HYPERTENSION

What is the best type of exercise for a particular patient/athlete?

The 36th Bethesda Conference provided recommendations for athletes with cardiovascular or structural abnormalities to lessen the risk of sudden cardiac death or disease progression (Table 6.2) [27]. Sports were categorized into two general types: dynamic (producing a volume load on the LV) and static (producing a pressure load on the LV) [33]. Sports are further classified according to level of intensity: low, medium, and high, and also as to whether there is a contact/collision component (Figure 6.1). Physicians can use Figure 6.1 as a guide to help to determine whether it is reasonably safe to recommend participation in competitive sports for athletes with HTN or to suggest activities suitable for cross-training to keep athletes active and aerobically conditioned during work-up or treatment. Such decisions must be individualized.

Many physical activities involve both static and dynamic components. For example, distance running has low static and high dynamic demands, while water skiing has prin-

Table 6.2 Recommendations of the 36th Bethesda Conference for hypertension in athletes (with permission from [27]).

1. Before individuals commence training for competitive athletics, they should undergo careful assessment of BP and those with initially high levels (above 140/90 mmHg) should have out-of-office measurements to exclude isolated office "white-coat hypertension". Those with pre-hypertension (120/80 mmHg up to 139/89 mmHg) should be encouraged to modify lifestyle but should not be restricted from physical activity. Those with sustained hypertension should have echocardiography. Left ventricular hypertrophy (LVH) beyond that seen with "athletes' heart" should limit participation until BP is normalized by appropriate drug therapy.
2. The presence of stage 1 hypertension in the absence of target organ damage including LVH or concomitant heart disease should not limit the eligibility for any competitive sport. Once having begun a training program, the hypertensive athlete should have BP re-measured every 2–4 months (or more frequently, if indicated) to monitor the impact of exercise.
3. Athletes with more severe hypertension (stage 2), even without evidence of target organ damage such as LVH, should be restricted, particularly from high static sports (classes IIIA to IIIC), until their hypertension is controlled by either lifestyle modification or drug therapy.
4. All drugs being taken must be registered with appropriate governing bodies to obtain a therapeutic exemption.
5. When hypertension coexists with another cardiovascular disease, eligibility for participation in competitive athletics is usually based on the type and severity of the associated condition.

cipally high static and low dynamic demands, and rowing has both high static and dynamic demands [33]. Thus, sports can be classified (Figure 6.1) as IIIC (high static, high dynamic), IIB (moderate static, moderate dynamic), IA (low static, low dynamic), etc. For example, an athlete with stage 2 HTN would be advised to avoid sports classified as IIIA, IIIB, and IIIC but may be able to participate in a IA sport until evaluation is complete and the BP is under control. Many athletes now use heavy resistance weight training (high static and low dynamic demand) for increasing strength and power in sports that do not impose heavy static demands during competition (e.g. tennis, basketball) [33]. It may be possible to modify such training regimens to reduce the cardiovascular demands to an acceptable level.

Asymptomatic individuals with controlled HTN and no cardiovascular disease or renal complications may participate in exercise or competitive athletics but should be monitored closely [7]. Preliminary peak or symptom-limited exercise testing may be warranted, especially for men over 45 and women over 55 years of age who are planning a vigorous exercise program (i.e. ≥60% maximum oxygen consumption or, to make it more clinically relevant, exercise that produces breathlessness so that patients cannot carry on a conversation: "can't talk exercise"). A stress test should be performed in patients who are symptomatic (i.e. exertional chest pain or dyspnea), whose BP exceeds 180/90 mmHg, or when there is known metabolic disease (e.g. diabetes mellitus). During the evaluation and management phase, it is reasonable for the majority of patients to begin moderate intensity exercise (40–60% of maximum age predicted heart rate) such as walking or other "talk exercise" [7].

TREATMENT OF THE HYPERTENSIVE ATHLETE

Healthcare providers should be aware that recreational, scholastic, and professional athletes have unique physiologic and psychological attributes. Even though they can look and feel fit, they can still have HTN and must periodically have their BP measured. Since regular physical

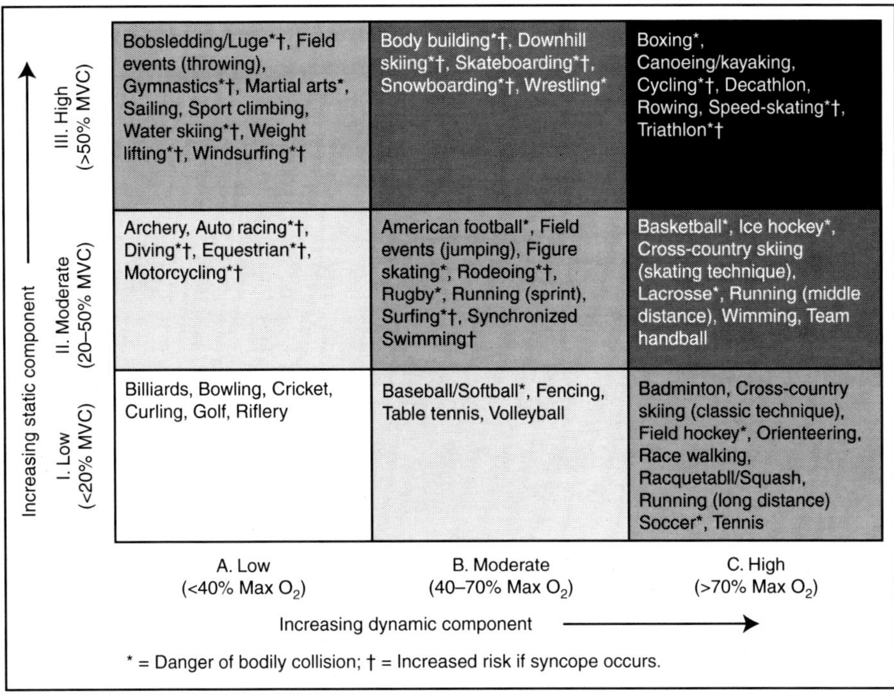

Figure 6.1 Classification of sports. This classification is based on peak static and dynamic components achieved during competition. It should be noted, however, that higher values may be reached during training. The increasing dynamic component is defined in terms of the estimated percent of maximal oxygen uptake (MaxO$_2$) achieved and results in an increasing cardiac output. The increasing static component is related to the estimated percent of maximal voluntary contraction (MVC) reached and results in an increasing blood pressure load. The lowest total cardiovascular demands (cardiac output and blood pressure) are shown at the bottom left (white) and the highest at the top right of the figure (black). Pale gray, mid gray and dark gray depict low moderate, moderate, and high moderate total cardiovascular demands (with permission from [33]).

activity reduces BP and has a wide range of other physical and psychological benefits, one of the goals of healthcare providers should be to keep athletes as active as possible.

What lifestyle modifications are most germane to the athlete with hypertension?

Untreated HTN in athletes may be accompanied by a varying degree of limitation in exercise performance [34]. Healthy lifestyle behaviors may not eliminate the need for antihypertensives but may reduce the amount of medication needed to achieve BP control (Table 6.3). The most effective dietary and lifestyle changes in athletes include losing weight and decreasing sodium intake [35], especially by reducing processed food intake. These lifestyle changes are particularly important for high-risk individuals such as African Americans, the elderly, and those with diabetes mellitus. Also of potential importance are increased potassium intake, decreased alcohol consumption, avoidance of tobacco (in any form) and drugs of abuse (especially sympathomimetics such as cocaine or ephedra). Other drugs to avoid include androgens, anabolic steroids, and growth hormone. The athlete (with hypertension or otherwise) often has a need for NSAID therapy and, if so, it should be undertaken cautiously at the lowest therapeutic dose possible. For athletes in static sports, performing regular aerobic exercise is desirable.

Table 6.3 Lifestyle modifications to reduce blood pressure in athletes.

Reduce sodium intake: African Americans, elderly, diabetics
Increase potassium intake: endurance athletes
Weight loss
Reduce alcohol intake
No tobacco (any form)
Avoid NSAIDs, herbals, sympathomimetics, human growth hormone, anabolic steroids
Relaxation techniques: meditation, yoga, tai chi
Light aerobic exercise

What are the best medications for the treatment of hypertension in the athlete from an efficacy and side-effect point of view?

The most common and best tolerated medications used for the treatment of HTN in athletes are vasodilators [36], especially ACE inhibitors or angiotensin receptor blockers (ARBs). These agents have no major adverse effects on energy metabolism and do not impair maximum oxygen uptake [37]. ARBs produce similar BP-lowering and hemodynamic patterns as ACE inhibitors but have fewer side-effects, especially cough and angioedema. In older athletes and African Americans, calcium channel blockers or low-dose thiazide diuretics are useful alternatives. Combination therapy may be needed in a few athletes; in that regard, the effectiveness of ACE inhibitors and ARBs is markedly improved by the addition of a thiazide diuretic or a calcium channel blocker. Some athletes benefit from β-blockade but these agents are banned in certain precision sports. Older agents such as alpha methyldopa and hydralazine are rarely used [38, 39].

Side-effects in athletes are generally similar to those seen in non-athletes. Neither ACE inhibitors nor ARBs should be given to women of child-bearing potential [31]. There have been anecdotal reports of postural hypotension after intense exercise in patients taking ACE inhibitors, so an adequate cool-down period is recommended [36]. Both antihypertensive potency and potassium-sparing effect of ACE inhibitors may be increased when they are taken concomitantly with NSAIDs [40]. Possible side-effects of thiazides within the first month include increased urinary loss of potassium and magnesium that can lead to muscle cramps and cardiac arrhythmias, particularly in warm weather. Initial hypovolemia and orthostatic hypotension can occur with thiazides but beyond the first week of treatment, plasma and extracellular volume tend to return to pre-treatment levels and the sustained BP-lowering effects are attributable to systemic arteriolar dilation [41].

Banned agents

The World Anti-Doping Agency, the US Olympic Committee, and the National Collegiate Athletic Association (NCAA) have banned the use of some antihypertensive medications [42]. Beta-blockers are banned in certain precision sports such as archery, shooting, diving, and figure skating [42]. Sports regulatory bodies have banned the use of all diuretics because they can mask the presence of anabolic steroids, so thiazides cannot be used by elite athletes who must undergo drug testing [42].

SUMMARY

Regular physical activity and training are associated with reductions in BP via mechanisms thought primarily to reflect neurochemical and structural changes that reduce peripheral vascular resistance yet elevated BP is one of the most common abnormalities found during the pre-participation physical evaluation of athletes. Hypertension remains the most common cardiovascular condition encountered in athletic populations, so all athletes require screening for HTN. Because athletes often have "white coat HTN", BP recordings outside the office are also necessary. The 36th Bethesda Conference classified sports according to their varying physiologic demands and provided specific recommendations for the evaluation, treatment and sport participation of athletes with HTN. In general, ACE inhibitors and other vasodilators are the medications of choice for active and athletic patients because of their limited interference with cardiovascular conditioning. Other agents can be used but some sports governing bodies proscribe the use of certain antihypertensive medications for elite athletes.

CASE STUDY

A 16-year-old, 6′ 4″, 210 pound African-American male presents for a PPE for basketball. His family history is positive for HTN in his father and his social history reveals no pattern of substance abuse. General physical examination is unremarkable except for BP of 144/94 mmHg in both arms (confirmed by repeat measurements 5 minutes later). He was told to measure morning and evening BP at home and he returned 2 weeks later with average home BPs of 128/82 mmHg.

What are the issues that this case raises for practitioners and what should practitioners do to evaluate and manage elevated BP readings in athletes?
His office BP values placed him in the 99th percentile for his gender, age, and height yet his final diagnosis was "white coat HTN". He was counseled about lifestyle modifications, was allowed to participate in basketball without medication, and did well on follow-up.

REFERENCES

1. Lehmann M, Durr H, Merkelbach H, Schmid A. Hypertension and sports activities: institutional experience. *Clin Cardiol* 1990; 13:197–208.
2. Whelton SP, Chin A, Xin X, He J. Effect of aerobic exercise on blood pressure: a meta-analysis of randomized, controlled trials. *Ann Intern Med* 2002; 136:493–503.
3. Cornelissen VA, Fagard RH. Effects of endurance training on blood pressure, blood pressure-regulating mechanisms, and cardiovascular risk factors. *Hypertension* 2005; 46:667–675.
4. Tanji JL. Tracking of elevated blood pressure values in adolescent athletes at 1-year follow-up. *Am J Dis Child* 1991; 145:665–667.
5. O'Connor FG, Meyering CD, Patel R, Oriscello RP. Hypertension, athletes, and the sports physician: implications of JNC VII, the Fourth Report, and the 36th Bethesda Conference Guidelines. *Curr Sports Med Rep* 2007; 6:80–84.
6. Caspersen CJ, Powell KE, Christenson GM. Physical activity, exercise, and physical fitness: definitions and distinctions for health-related research. *Public Health Rep* 1985; 100:126–131.
7. Pescatello LS, Franklin BA, Fagard R, Farquhar WB, Kelley GA, Ray CA. American College of Sports Medicine position stand. Exercise and hypertension. *Med Sci Sports Exerc* 2004; 36:533–553.
8. Chobanian AV, Bakris GL, Black HR *et al*. The seventh report of the Joint National Committee on Prevention, Detection, Evaluation, and Treatment of High Blood Pressure: the JNC-7 report. *JAMA* 2003; 289:2560–2572.
9. Williams PT. Physical fitness and activity as separate heart disease risk factors: a meta-analysis. *Med Sci Sports Exerc* 2001; 33:754–761.
10. Williams PT. Vigorous exercise, fitness and incident hypertension, high cholesterol, and diabetes. *Med Sci Sports Exerc* 2008; 40:998–1006.
11. Blair SN, Cheng Y, Holder JS. Is physical activity or physical fitness more important in defining health benefits? *Med Sci Sports Exerc* 2001; 33:S379–S399; discussion S419–S420.

12. Blair SN, Jackson AS. Physical fitness and activity as separate heart disease risk factors: a meta-analysis. *Med Sci Sports Exerc* 2001; 33:762–764.

13. Williams NH, Hendry M, France B, Lewis R, Wilkinson C. Effectiveness of exercise-referral schemes to promote physical activity in adults: systematic review. *Br J Gen Pract* 2007; 57:979–986.

14. Ignarro LJ, Balestrieri ML, Napoli C. Nutrition, physical activity, and cardiovascular disease: an update. *Cardiovasc Res* 2007; 73:326–340.

15. Cornelissen VA, Fagard RH. Effect of resistance training on resting blood pressure: a meta-analysis of randomized controlled trials. *J Hypertens* 2005; 23:251–259.

16. Hanson P, Andrea BE. Treatment of hypertension in athletes. In: Delee J, Drez D, Stanitski CL (eds). *Orthopaedic Sports Medicine: Principles and Practice*. Saunders, Baltimore, 1994, pp 307–319.

17. Schmid A, Schmidt-Trucksass A, Huonker M et al. Catecholamines response of high performance wheelchair athletes at rest and during exercise with autonomic dysreflexia. *Int J Sports Med* 2001; 22:2–7.

18. Kouidi E, Fahadidou-Tsiligiroglou A, Tassoulas E, Deligiannis A, Coats A. White coat hypertension detected during screening of male adolescent athletes. *Am J Hypertens* 1999; 12:223–226.

19. Pelliccia A. Athlete's heart and hypertrophic cardiomyopathy. *Curr Cardiol Rep* 2000; 2:166–171.

20. Dlin RA, Dotan R, Inbar O, Rotstein A, Jacobs I, Karlsson J. Exaggerated systolic blood pressure response to exercise in a water polo team. *Med Sci Sports Exerc* 1984; 16:294–298.

21. Mahmud A, Feely J. Spurious systolic hypertension of youth: fit young men with elastic arteries. *Am J Hypertens* 2003; 16:229–232.

22. Hulsen HT, Nijdam ME, Bos WJ et al. Spurious systolic hypertension in young adults: prevalence of high brachial systolic blood pressure and low central pressure and its determinants. *J Hypertens* 2006; 24:1027–1032.

23. Nelson TF, Wechsler H. Alcohol and college athletes. *Med Sci Sports Exerc* 2001; 33:43–47.

24. Kaplan NM, Lieberman E. *Clinical Hypertension*, 6th edition. Williams & Wilkins, Baltimore, 1994.

25. Baker RH, Ende J. Confounders of auscultatory blood pressure measurement. *J Gen Intern Med* 1995; 10:223–231.

26. Hall WD. Pitfalls in the diagnosis and management of systolic hypertension. *South Med J* 2000; 93:256–259.

27. Kaplan NM, Gidding SS, Pickering TG, Wright JT Jr. Task Force 5: systemic hypertension. *J Am Coll Cardiol* 2005; 45:1346–1348.

28. Bates B. *A Guide to the Physical Examination and History Taking*, 5th edition. Lippincott Williams & Wilkins, Philadelphia, PA, 1991.

29. Rahiala E, Tikanoja T. Suspicion of aortic coarctation in an outpatient clinic: how should blood pressure measurements be performed? *Clin Physiol* 2001; 21:100–104.

30. The fourth report on the diagnosis, evaluation, and treatment of high blood pressure in children and adolescents. *Pediatrics* 2004; 114:555–576.

31. Rangarajan U, Kochar MS. Hypertension in women. *WMJ* 2000; 99:65–70.

32. Maron BJ. Structural features of the athlete heart as defined by echocardiography. *J Am Coll Cardiol* 1986; 7:190–203.

33. Mitchell JH, Haskell W, Snell P, Van Camp SP. Task Force 8: classification of sports. *J Am Coll Cardiol* 2005; 45:1364–1367.

34. Missault L, Duprez D, de Buyzere M, de Backer G, Clement D. Decreased exercise capacity in mild essential hypertension: non-invasive indicators of limiting factors. *J Hum Hypertens* 1992; 6:151–155.

35. Kojuri J, Rahimi R. Effect of "no added salt diet" on blood pressure control and 24 hour urinary sodium excretion in mild to moderate hypertension. *BMC Cardiovasc Disord* 2007; 7:34.

36. Niedfeldt MW. Managing hypertension in athletes and physically active patients. *Am Fam Physician* 2002; 66:445–452.

37. Chick TW, Halperin AK, Gacek EM. The effect of antihypertensive medications on exercise performance: a review. *Med Sci Sports Exerc* 1988; 20:447–454.

38. Chobanian AV, Bakris GL, Black HR et al. Seventh report of the Joint National Committee on Prevention, Detection, Evaluation, and Treatment of High Blood Pressure. *Hypertension* 2003; 42:1206–1252.

39. Handler J. Managing chronic severe hypertension in pregnancy. *J Clin Hypertens (Greenwich)* 2006; 8:738–743.

40. Gifford RW Jr. Antihypertensive therapy. Angiotensin-converting enzyme inhibitors, angiotensin II receptor antagonists, and calcium antagonists. *Med Clin North Am* 1997; 81:1319–1333.

41. Hughes AD. How do thiazide and thiazide-like diuretics lower blood pressure? *J Renin Angiotensin Aldosterone Syst* 2004; 5:155–160.
42. WADA. The World Anti-Doping Code. *The 2010 Prohibited List. International Standard.* http://www.wada-ama.org/Documents/World_Anti-Doping_Program/WADP-Prohibited-list/ WADA_Prohibited_List_2010_EN.pdf.

7

Management of hypertensive emergencies

S. U. Rehman, D. G. Vidt, J. Basile

BACKGROUND

Even though 1% of hypertensive patients will present with a hypertensive crisis [1], they account for up to 25% of all emergency department visits [2, 3]. Patients with hypertensive crises may present with a range of blood pressures, varied clinical symptoms and the presence or absence of target organ involvement. Early triage in the emergency department is critical to identify those individuals who may require more aggressive management in the emergency room or admission for parenteral therapy. This review will focus on patients with severe hypertension (hypertensive urgencies) or those deemed to have a true hypertensive emergency.

WHAT DISTINGUISHES A HYPERTENSIVE URGENCY FROM A HYPERTENSIVE EMERGENCY?

Traditionally, hypertensive crises have been classified as either an emergency or an urgency [4]. A *hypertensive emergency* is a severe and often sudden onset elevation of blood pressure (BP) associated with acute and often progressive target organ dysfunction and is a true medical emergency. A hypertensive emergency requires immediate BP reduction (not necessarily to normal levels though) with intravenous (IV) therapy if end-organ damage is to be limited [1, 5].

Patients with hypertensive emergencies present with acute and ongoing target organ damage. Cerebral infarction is the most common presentation (24.5%), followed by acute pulmonary edema (22.5%), hypertensive encephalopathy (16.3%), acute congestive heart failure (14.3%), acute myocardial infarction or unstable angina pectoris (12.0%), acute intracerebral or subarachnoid hemorrhage (4.5%), eclampsia (4.5%) and aortic dissection (2.0%) [3].

Hypertensive emergencies are frequently defined based on the severity of the BP elevation (systolic BP in excess of 200 mmHg or a diastolic BP greater than 120 mmHg), but it is important to note that it is *not* the degree of BP elevation but rather the clinical presentation of the patient that is the basis for the emergency. Patients with only moderate elevations of BP may also present as an emergency with acute and ongoing target organ damage. For example, a BP of 160/100

Shakaib U. Rehman, MD, FACP, FAACH, Chief of Primary Care, Associate Professor of Medicine, Ralph H. Johnson VA Medical Center, Medical University of South Carolina, Charleston, South Carolina, USA.

Donald G. Vidt, MD, Emeritus Chairman/Consultant, Department of Hypertension and Nephrology, Cleveland Clinic, Cleveland, Ohio, USA.

Jan Basile, MD, Professor of Medicine, Seinsheimer Cardiovascular Health Program, Division of General Internal Medicine/Geriatrics, Medical University of South Carolina, Research Associate, Primary Care Service Line, Ralph H. Johnson VA Medical Center, Charleston, South

Table 7.1 Clinical situations representing hypertensive emergencies (adapted with permission from [17]).

1. Hypertensive encephalopathy
2. Malignant hypertension: elevated blood pressure with papilledema (some cases)
3. Intracranial hemorrhage (intracerebral or subarachnoid) or acute atherothrombotic brain infarction
4. Acute coronary syndromes (unstable angina/myocardial infarction)
5. Acute left ventricular failure with pulmonary edema
6. Aortic dissection
7. Rapidly progressive renal failure, for example systemic vasculitis including scleroderma crisis
8. Eclampsia
9. Severe postoperative arterial bleeding
10. Head trauma
11. Less common situations:
    - Pheochromocytoma crisis,
    - Tyramine interaction with MAO inhibitors,
    - Sympathomimetic drugs like phencyclidine, LSD, cocaine, or phenylpropanolamine,
    - Rebound hypertension following the sudden withdrawal of antihypertensive agents such as clonidine or β-blockers

mmHg in a 68-year-old man with abdominal pain from progressive aortic dissection or a woman in her third trimester of pregnancy with proteinuria, edema, and convulsions (eclampsia) represent true hypertensive emergencies despite the modest elevation in BP. In contrast, a 60-year-old female with a BP of 210/120 mmHg and no evidence of target organ damage does not require hospitalization or aggressive lowering of BP as long as timely out-patient follow-up is available and therapy has been begun and it is clear that the patient will be compliant with the regimen. Patients with a true hypertensive emergency are most appropriately treated with parenteral medications in an intensive care unit setting or at a minimum in a monitored bed. Table 7.1 shows the clinical situations most often presenting as hypertensive emergencies.

Severe BP elevation (so-called "hypertensive urgencies")

This is defined by the Seventh Report of the Joint National Committee on Prevention, Detection, Evaluation, and Treatment of High BP as severe elevations in BP without progressive target organ dysfunction [4]. In other instances, it has been defined as patients with diastolic BP of greater than 110 to 120 mmHg or systolic BP of greater than 180 mmHg [6]. Patients may present with severe headache, anxiety, shortness of breath and/or epistaxis [4]. Some of these patients may have signs of chronic target organ damage, such as retinal hemorrhages and exudates, left ventricular hypertrophy, or chronic renal insufficiency but with stable renal function. It is the absence of progressively worsening hypertensive target organ damage, however, that differentiates these patients from hypertensive emergencies. There is currently no evidence showing the benefit of acutely lowering BP in asymptomatic patients with severe hypertension [4, 6]; in fact, there is some evidence to suggest that rapid lowering of BP in some such patients is associated with adverse outcomes [7, 8]. Unfortunately, the term "urgency" has been ingrained in the literature and has led to overly aggressive treatment for asymptomatic hypertension (with sometimes adverse consequences) in emergency departments throughout the world, often with one or more parenteral medications given to rapidly normalize BP [8, 9]. Even the oral loading doses of antihypertensive agents can have cumulative hypotensive effects, sometimes following discharge from the emergency department [4]. A recent study found that less than one-fifth of the patients seen in an emergency room with a presumed hypertensive crisis met defined criteria for this diagnosis and the

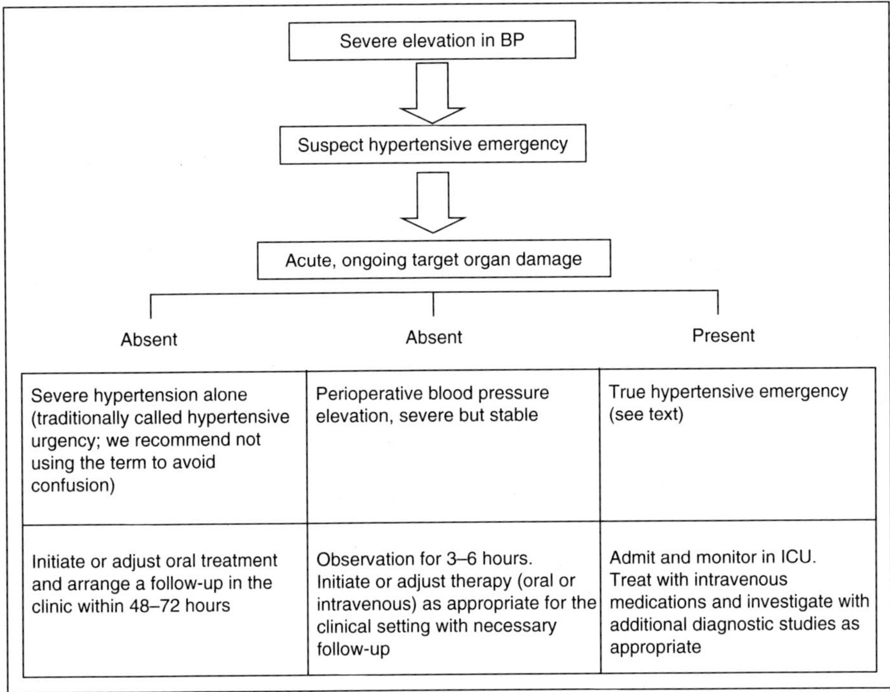

Figure 7.1 Triage of suspected hypertensive emergencies.

medical management was considered appropriate in less than half of the occurrences [2]. In fact, most of these patients are non-compliant or inadequately treated hypertensives and do not require hospital admission or acute lowering of their BP. In most instances, such patients can be safely treated as out-patients with oral antihypertensive medications.

We recommend dropping the term 'hypertensive urgency' since this label has caused unnecessary over-treatment and harm to patients when clinicians react to BP numbers rather than to the clinical situation [9, 10]. We suggest that *hypertensive urgencies*, except for perioperative hypertension (discussed later), should better be classified as *severe hypertension* without ongoing target organ damage. We will not be using the term "urgency" in the remainder of the chapter. Despite its widespread use, we also recommend not using the term "malignant hypertension" (with its associated papilledema) due to the lack of evidence supporting the definition as well as the vagueness of this terminology. Physicians should therefore treat the patient and assess for ongoing target organ damage rather than act on the severity of BP elevation (*treating the patient rather than their numbers*). The appropriate differentiation of these two forms of hypertensive crises is extremely important if better outcomes are to be realized in patients with very high BP. Figure 7.1 shows an algorithm by which patients with severe elevations in BP can be promptly triaged for admission to receive parenteral or, where appropriate, out-patient oral therapy.

WHICH CONCOMITANT ILLNESSES AND MEDICATIONS/RECREATIONAL DRUGS CAN TRIGGER HYPERTENSIVE CRISES?

The vast majority of patients presenting with a hypertensive crisis have a prior diagnosis of hypertension and have been prescribed antihypertensive agents [11] However, in many of these patients, BP control prior to presentation was inadequate [11]. The lack of a primary care physician has also been associated with a higher likelihood for presenting as a hypertensive emergency [12]. One study found that 50% of patients presenting to an emergency department with a hypertensive emergency were not compliant with their antihypertensive medication regimen in the preceding week [12]. Illicit drug use (amphetamines, cocaine, and phencyclidine) has been reported to be a major risk factor for the development of a hypertensive emergency. [13] Low socio-economic status with poor access to healthcare, drug and alcohol abuse, oral contraceptive use, and cigarette smoking may also increase one's risk of presenting as a hypertensive emergency [13]. It is important to note that all of these are preventable causes of hypertensive emergencies. Providing access to and encouraging patients to have good follow-up with their primary care physicians as well as complying with their antihypertensive regimen improves BP control and reduces the frequency of severe BP elevations.

WHAT CONSTITUTES AN APPROPRIATE CLINICAL EVALUATION OF A HYPERTENSIVE CRISIS?

Patients presenting with severe elevation of BP should be triaged early to assess the level of target end organ damage [14], keeping in mind that therapy may need to be initiated before the evaluation and work-up are completed. Physicians should complete a quick and targeted history and a focused physical examination along with ordering laboratory studies sufficient to establish the level of renal function, the presence of electrolyte abnormalities (e.g. hypokalemia), and the anemia status. The algorithm in Figure 7.1 aids in the early identification of those hypertensive emergencies that require immediate admission/prompt attention. The history should include questioning for symptoms related to ongoing target organ damage such as headaches, changes in mentation, seizures, focal weakness, visual change, chest pain, shortness of breath, and new or worsening peripheral edema. Taking a careful history regarding antihypertensive medications with dosing, compliance with medication regimens, the time from last dose and prior control rates is of particular importance. Acute withdrawal of hypertensive medications, such as β-blockers and high-dose clonidine, may cause severe rebound elevations in BP. The use of any prescribed, over-the-counter medications, herbal preparations, or illicit substances, especially cocaine, should be documented. Use of sympathomimetic medications such as decongestants, anticholinergic medications including antidepressants, amphetamines, and alcohol ingestion may cause severe elevations in BP [15].

Blood pressure should be measured in both arms using a standard sphygmomanometer. It is very important to measure BP with an appropriately sized cuff in that cuffs too small for a particular arm size can be associated with erroneously elevated BP readings. Automated BP monitoring devices may not be accurate in patients with very high BP readings making a crosscheck of BP with a standard sphygmomanometer important. All patients should have a funduscopic examination carefully looking for hemorrhages, exudates, and papilledema. A cardiovascular exam should document radial, femoral, and carotid pulses. Pulse deficits should raise the suspicion for aortic dissection. A quick neurological examination including mental status should be carried out. Headache and altered mental status are findings indicative of hypertensive encephalopathy. Focal neurologic findings are uncommon in hypertensive encephalopathy and more often suggest a cerebrovascular accident to have occurred. The sudden onset of a severe occipital headache, with or without neurologic findings, should raise for consideration the possibility of a subarachnoid hemorrhage.

Clinical evaluation should guide further diagnostic testing. Very few studies have assessed the prognostic value of abnormal laboratory findings in patients with asymptomatic severe hypertension [6, 16]. The Seventh Report of the Joint National Committee on the Prevention, Detection, Evaluation, and Treatment of High Blood Pressure (JNC-7) recommends a complete blood cell count including a peripheral smear to look for the presence of schistocytes indicative of microangiopathic hemolytic anemia, and a metabolic profile evaluating electrolytes, blood urea nitrogen, serum creatinine, and urinalysis. If the urinalysis reveals proteinuria, it should be compared to a previous urinanalysis (if available) to determine if the proteinuria is new, worsening, or unchanged from baseline. New or worsening proteinuria may signify acute kidney injury. Red blood cell (RBC) and/or RBC casts in a urinalysis also point to an active glomerular process. An electrocardiogram should be performed to rule out cardiac ischemia. There is no evidence on the benefits of obtaining a chest radiograph in asymptomatic patients [17], except in patients who have symptoms suggesting pulmonary edema. A computed tomographic (CT) scan of the brain should be considered in patients with an acute change in mental status or acute neurological signs and symptoms suggestive of cerebral encephalopathy, ischemia or hemorrhage. A contrast-enhanced CT scan or magnetic resonance imaging (MRI) of the chest should be obtained if aortic dissection is suspected (severe chest pain, unequal pulses, and widened mediastinum).

Once the patient is stable, an investigation into any secondary causes of hypertension should be undertaken. While a secondary cause will be identified in many Caucasian patients presenting with a hypertensive emergency (especially those under the age of 30 years), a secondary cause is less frequently found in patients of African-American descent [18].

WHAT IS THE APPROPRIATE MANAGEMENT OF PATIENTS WITH SEVERE HYPERTENSION (SO CALLED HYPERTENSIVE URGENCY)?

Patients with *severe hypertension* should be treated with oral medications to lower the BP gradually over 24 to 48 h. Two or more antihypertensive agents, one of which is a diuretic or a calcium channel blocker, may be started together. In the choice of agents to begin therapy, with one approach is to resume a prior regimen if it had been well-tolerated. Another approach recently suggested is for patients with *severe hypertension* presenting to an emergency room to be given an initial 30-minute rest period. In a recent study where this approach was employed about one-third of patients had a meaningful BP response to rest alone (systolic BP <180 mmHg and diastolic BP <110 mmHg with at least a 20/10 mmHg drop in BP). In the other two-thirds of patients in this study whose BP did not respond to rest, 68% had a satisfactory and safe BP response to oral antihypertensive drug treatment (perindopril, amlodipine, or labetalol) over a 2-hour average follow-up period [19].

In the past, many patients with *severe hypertension* were prescribed short-acting nifedipine, whether given by mouth or sublingually [20, 21]. This practice, however, has been associated with occasional precipitous falls in BP leading to acute ischemic stroke and myocardial infarction and has fallen out of favor over the last several years [22]. The role of pain, anxiety and panic attacks should be recognized when managing patients with severe BP elevation with or without acute target organ damage, since these conditions may also significantly elevate the BP. Analgesics and anxiolytics should be utilized in these situations, as indicated [23].

There is no need to normalize BP in the patient with *severe hypertension* before discharge since there is no evidence that these patients are at risk for an immediate vascular event (e.g. stroke, myocardial infarction) [4, 6, 24]. It is important to appreciate that most of these patients have had an elevated BP for some time and their autoregulatory processes have already been set at a higher BP level. Patients can be discharged from the emergency room even if their BP is still elevated as long as a follow-up appointment with a qualified practitioner is in place (*see* Figure 7.1). Follow-up is very important as some patients may view treatment provided in the emergency room setting as "curative", with the consequences and chronic effects of uncontrolled hypertension then going poorly appreciated. Long-term follow-up is essential to make sure patients receive proper treatment, assessment of BP control, monitoring of adherence to medication, and education about lifestyle modifications such as smoking cessation, sodium restriction, exercise, a proper diet, and weight loss.

HOW ARE PATIENTS SUSPECTED OF HAVING A HYPERTENSIVE EMERGENCY BEST MANAGED INITIALLY?

Therapeutic decisions are based upon the presence of acute and progressive target organ damage and *not* solely on the level of BP. The primary goal of treatment is to prevent or limit target organ damage. Therapy should be initiated immediately for rapid BP reduction, often before the results of all initial laboratory studies are available, preferably with a titrable, short acting IV antihypertensive agent. Intramuscular and sublingual routes should be avoided due to the time-wise unpredictability of their pharmacodynamic response [25]. Patients with a true hypertensive emergency require immediate admission to an intensive care or monitored bed for continuous BP monitoring as they are being given parenteral therapy [26]. It should be emphasized that the goal is not to lower BP to normal ranges, as this may cause an even more rapid deterioration in renal function than is usually the case and/or precipitate a cardiac or cerebral event [4, 27]. The initial goal of therapy is to reduce mean arterial BP (MAP) by no more than 25% below the pre-treatment level within the first two h of treatment. Over the next 2 to 6 hours, BP should be reduced slowly toward 160/100 mmHg. If this level of BP is well tolerated and the patient is clinically stable, further gradual reductions towards a normal BP can be implemented over the next 24 to 48 hours. Conversion from parenteral to oral therapy for the patient with a hypertensive emergency is best begun early in the course of treatment. In so doing it can be determined whether oral therapy will "hold" the patient at an acceptable BP level prior to their being discharged. Some patients, however, with a hypertensive emergency (*under special circumstances*) require specific treatment strategies, which are described later.

WHAT PARENTERAL THERAPIES ARE AVAILABLE FOR TREATMENT OF HYPERTENSIVE EMERGENCIES?

Hypertensive emergency treatment recommendations are based mostly on consensus opinion [4, 6, 24, 28] since there are no randomized controlled trials (RCTs) showing that specific anti-hypertensive drugs reduce mortality or morbidity in these patients. Also, there are insufficient outcome-based studies to determine which drug is most effective in reducing mortality and morbidity [29, 30]. There are, however, some minor differences in the degree of BP reduction that occurs when one class of antihypertensive drug is compared to another [6, 29, 31].

Table 7.2 lists agents commonly utilized for the management of the hypertensive emergency. When the desired BP level is achieved, oral agents can be started to facilitate tapering of the parenteral agent as well as preventing rebound hypertension. Loop diuretics should not be used initially in the treatment of patients with a hypertensive emergency except in patients where there is evidence of volume overload (such as those with congestive heart failure (CHF), cirrhosis, or nephrotic syndrome), as many of these patients are often intravascularly volume contracted due to pressure natriuresis [4, 28]. In that regard, fluid replacement has been observed to lower BP and improve renal function in a subset of patients with severe hypertension and evidence of hypovolemia. Later in the course of treatment, sodium and volume retention may be caused by many of the same parenteral agents used for treatment, which may lead to resistance to further BP reduction (tachyphylaxis). Here, loop diuretics may also be necessary if further BP reduction is to occur [28].

HOW ARE SPECIAL SITUATION PATIENTS MANAGED WHEN THEY PRESENT WITH A HYPERTENSIVE EMERGENCY?

Aortic dissection

The initial goal of medical therapy in patients with aortic dissection is to decrease both systemic BP and the force of left ventricular contraction. Patients with aortic dissection

Table 7.2 Parenteral drugs for treatment of hypertensive emergencies (modified from JNC-7).

Drug	Dose	Onset of action	Duration of action	Adverse effects	Special indication	Special caution
Sodium nitroprusside [42]	0.25–10 µg/kg/ min as IV infusion	Immediate	1–2 min	Nausea, vomiting, muscle spasm, sweating, thiocyanate and cyanide intoxication Extended use for periods >3 days may result in thiocyanate toxicity	Most hypertensive emergencies	*Raised intracranial pressure*: cerebral blood flow may decrease in a dose dependent manner *Azotemia*: toxic metabolite may accumulate *Eclampsia*: as drug crosses placenta *Special equipment*: requires light-resistant equipment
Nitroglycerine	5–100 µg/min as IV infusion	2–5 min	5–10 min	Headache, vomiting, methemoglobinemia, tolerance with prolonged use	Coronary ischemia, acute LV failure, postoperative hypertension	Not first-line in other situations due to unpredictable antihypertensive effects and development of tolerance
Fenoldopam [43]	0.1–0.3 µg/kg/ min IV infusion	<5 min	30 min	Reflex tachycardia, hypokalemia, headache, flushing, nausea, increased intraocular pressure and ECG changes	Most hypertensive emergencies, comparable to nitroprusside Requires intra-arterial monitoring May be the drug of choice in those with renal insufficiency	Never administer as IV bolus Caution with glaucoma

Table 7.2 Continued.

Drug	Dose	Onset of action	Duration of action	Adverse effects	Special indication	Special caution
Esmolol	250–500 µg/kg/min IV bolus, then 50–100 µg/kg/min by infusion May repeat	1–2 min	10–30 min	Hypotension, nausea, asthma, first-degree heart block, heart failure	Especially useful in aortic dissection, myocardial infarction, thyrotoxicosis and patients undergoing coronary artery bypass grafting [44]	Avoid in cocaine-induced hypertension
Enalaprilat	0.625–1.25 mg every 6 h IV	15–30 min	6–12 h	Precipitous fall in pressure in high renin states; variable response	Acute left ventricular failure. Drug of choice in scleroderma renal crisis	Contraindicated in bilateral renal artery stenosis and 2nd and 3rd trimester of pregnancy Avoid in acute myocardial infarction
Labetolol [44]	20–80 mg IV bolus every 10 min; 0.5–2 mg/min IV infusion	5–10 min	3–6 h	Vomiting, scalp tingling, burning sensation in throat, dizziness, nausea, heart block, orthostasis	Most hypertensive emergencies Particularly useful in eclampsia, pheochromocytoma and states of excess catecholamines	Contraindicated in heart block, bradycardia and bronchospasm Avoid in acute heart failure

Drug	Dose	Onset	Duration	Adverse effects	Indications	Special considerations
Nicardipine	5–15 mg/hr IV	5–10 min	30 min to 4 h	Tachycardia flushing, headache, local phlebitis	Most hypertensive emergencies Comparable to nitroprusside Reduces both cardiac and cerebral ischemia Dosage is not dependent on weight, allowing for ease of administration	Avoid in acute heart failure Caution with coronary ischemia
Hydralazine	10–20 mg IV; 10–40 mg IM	10–20 min IV; 20–30 min IM	1–4 h IV 4–6 h IM	Tachycardia flushing, headache, vomiting, aggravation of angina	Eclampsia	Contraindicated in coronary artery disease and aortic dissection
Clevidipine [45, 46]	1–2 mg/hr IV infusion (max. 16 mg/hr)	2–4 min	5–15 min	Tachycardia, headache, cardiac arrest, myocardial infarction	Perioperative hypertension	Contraindicated in patients with aortic stenosis and patients with allergy to soybeans, soy products, eggs, or egg products
Phentolamine	5–15 mg IV	1–2 min	3–10 min	Tachycardia, flushing, headache	Catecholamine excess, cocaine and amphetamine overdose, MAO inhibitor crisis	Contraindicated in pre-existing coronary artery disease

ECG = electrocardiogram; IM = intramuscular; IV = intravenous; LV = left ventricular; MAO = monoamine oxidase.

should have their systolic BP lowered to 100–120 mmHg or the lowest value that is tolerated without signs of hypoperfusion [32]. Blood pressure should be obtained in both arms in that aortic branch vessel occlusion may falsely lower BP in one arm or the other. Quite logically, the arm with the higher BP should be used for measurement. Adequate pain control is necessary to allay anxiety and to reduce sympathetic stimulation, which may importantly contribute to elevated BP. Beta-blockers such as esmolol, metoprolol or labetalol are first line agents because they have the desirable effect of reducing aortic shear stress. If BP pressure remains high after adequate β-blockade (at maximum dose or at heart rate <60 beats/min) additional vasodilator therapy such as nitroprusside can be added. Direct vasodilators, such as hydralazine and minoxidil, should not be used alone, because they can increase sympathetic drive, which increases the force of left ventricular ejection and risks further dissection. In patients for whom β-blockers are contraindicated, such as those who have severe asthma, rate lowering calcium-channel blockers with negative inotropic effects, such as diltiazem or verapamil can be given. Surgical consultation should be obtained as soon as possible.

Myocardial infarction

Intravenous nitrates are a practical choice in the presence of myocardial ischemia; nitrates have a modest BP lowering effect even as they improve coronary perfusion, and decrease left ventricular preload. Intravenous β-blockers are also handy agents in that they reduce both heart rate and BP and therein cut back myocardial oxygen demand. Pure vasodilators, such as hydralazine, should be eschewed because they can cause a reflex tachycardia that may itself increase myocardial oxygen demand [28].

Congestive heart failure

Patients with *de novo* systolic forms of HF tend to have lower BP due to a decreased left ventricular ejection fraction. A hypertensive emergency can in and of itself precipitate HF and can be treated with intravenous nitroglycerin or sodium nitroprusside [28]. Angiotensin converting enzyme (ACE) inhibitors have been used extensively because of their beneficial effects on both preload and afterload [33]; however enalaprilat is the only parenteral ACE inhibitor available. Diuretics should be used to the extent that volume overload is perceived as a contributing factor to the hypertension and/or for symptomatic relief. Of note, high-dose intravenous loop diuretic therapy can be accompanied by short-term (volume-independent) activation of the renin-angiotensin-aldosterone axis [34]. Intravenous nesiritide improves hemodynamic function in patients with decompensated HF and has a modest BP lowering effect; however, its use for antihypertensive purposes has not been formally studied and there remains some question as to adverse renal effects with its use [35].

Ischemic cerebrovascular accidents

An elevated BP is often seen shortly after a stroke and may be secondary to the stress of the event (increased intracranial pressure), pain, nausea, a distended bladder, and/or pre-existing hypertension. In many patients, BP falls spontaneously with rest, a peaceful environment, pain/nausea control and bladder emptying. Although severe hypertension may be viewed as an indication for immediate treatment in the setting of an ischemic cerebrovascular accident, no data specify the level(s) of hypertension that make emergency management imperative. From what data is available it would appear that a systolic BP level >180 mmHg should prompt treatment. Even as such, BP should be lowered cautiously (15 to 25% in the first day) since aggressive lowering of BP may result in worsening of the neurological status as ischemic areas of the brain are underperfused. Because no data support the administration of any specific antihypertensive agent in the setting of acute ischemic stroke, the treating physician should select medications for lowering blood pressure on a case-by-case basis; however, when parenteral therapy is indicated sodium nitroprusside, esmolol or labetalol have been recommended [36–38]. While nicardipine has been recommended, other CCBs have been linked to an increase in intracranial pressure, and therefore should be avoided in patients with brain injury [6].

Hemorrhagic cerebrovascular accidents

Theoretically, elevated BP may increase the risk of ongoing bleeding from ruptured small arteries and arterioles during the first hours; however, it has been difficult to determine with any certainty that elevated BP is a cause of greater hemorrhage. As such, prevention of complications by immediate reduction of BP is unproven in the instance of a hemorrhagic cerebrovascular accident [39]. Guidelines for BP control in patients with hemorrhagic stroke is similar to those for ischemic stroke; decreasing BP only when the systolic BP is greater than 180 mmHg or the mean arterial pressure is >130 mmHg. The optimal level of a patient's BP should be based on individual factors such as chronic hypertension, intracranial pressure values, patient age, presumed cause of hemorrhage, and the time since onset. Subarachnoid bleed is a form of cerebral hemorrhage where a specific drug the dihydropyridine CCB nimodipine is indicated to reduce cerebral artery spasm, which is a cause of delayed ischemic neurological deficits. Nimodipine has been shown to decrease the incidence of vasospasm and rebleeding after subarachnoid hemorrhage [36].

Pre-eclampsia

Hydralazine and labetalol have been the drugs of choice for the treatment of patients with severe BP elevation due to pre-eclempsia [28, 40]. Hydralazine is particularly popular among obstetricians because it does not inhibit uterine contractions and only minimally crosses the placental barrier. Hydralazine may cause significant dose-dependent reflex tachycardia – a side-effect that should be monitored closely. Labetalol has gradually replaced hydralazine as the most commonly used antihypertensive in the treatment of severe pre-eclampsia. It permits a more rapid and reliable reduction in blood pressure with fewer acute side-effects than is the case with hydralazine. Fetal risk with labetalol is low because fetal heart rate and uteroplacental blood flow change minimally with this compound. Calcium channel blockers, such as nifedipine and nicardipine, lower maternal blood pressure without compromising placental function and are useful second line agents [41]. Diuretics are used sparingly in this disease state in that these compounds may exacerbate the hypovolemia that marks this disease. ACE inhibitors and ARBs are contraindicated in pre-eclampsia as they are in the second and third trimester of pregnancy. While infusion of magnesium sulfate in these patients has been associated with a reduction in BP, the control of seizures, and a reduction in mortality, delivery of the fetus remains the most definitive therapy [4, 41].

Catecholamine crisis

Patients with pheochromocytoma usually have very high BP due to catecholamine induced α- receptor activation and are commonly treated with antihypertensive agents with α-blocking properties (e.g. phentolamine, administered intravenously). This might be accompanied by a β-blocker, as needed, if the patient develops tachycardia. Administration of β-blockers alone, in the presence of catecholamine excess, can lead to unopposed α-receptor activation with subsequent worsening of hypertension. Labetalol, a β-blocker with some α-antagonist properties, can be used under these circumstances. The drug phentolamine is often used in the patient with pheochromocytoma but such use should be under carefully controlled circumstances. Sympathomimetic drugs, such as phenylephrine, cocaine, and methamphetamine, can also cause a hypertensive crisis due to catecholamine excess. Labetalol or nitroprusside are treatments of choice.

Perioperative hypertension

BP elevation in the perioperative period may be the result of many factors including adrenergic stimulation from the surgical event, changes in intravascular volume, and/or pre/postoperative pain or anxiety. Patients with BP levels of 180/110 mmHg or greater either before or immediately after surgery have been found to be at a greater risk for cardiac events [4]. Most of these patients, however, have no signs of acute and ongoing target organ damage. Pre-operative hypertension is frequently a severe hypertension, not an emergency, as it typically does not involve end organ damage and there is usually adequate time to reduce the BP. BP should be lowered over the next 24 h to avoid cancellation of surgery as well as to improve perioperative cardiovascular outcomes. It may be appropriate to treat these patients with intravenous or oral agents depending upon the clinical situation. One important prevention strategy to minimize perioperative problems with BP control is that patients should be maintained on their out-patient oral antihypertensive regimen until surgery and these agents should be restarted as soon as possible after surgery, unless the patient is unable to resume oral intake in which case parenteral agents may be indicated. One preventive approach is to substitute long-acting preparations of the patient's long-term antihypertensive regimen starting, if possible, several days before surgery and to be given in the morning of the day of surgery.

SUMMARY

A hypertensive emergency is a severe and acute elevation in BP accompanied by progressive target organ damage (e.g. acute coronary syndromes, cerebral ischemia, pulmonary edema, renal failure, aortic dissection, or eclampsia). Patients with untreated hypertensive emergencies have a very high mortality and, as such, should be managed with intravenous medication(s) in an intensive care unit setting or monitored bed. While BP should be reduced within minutes to hours, the initial mean arterial pressure reduction should not be more than 20–25% of baseline BP to avoid hypoperfusion of vital organs. Once stable, patients should be investigated more thoroughly for an underlying cause of their hypertension. Proper education and appropriate follow-up should be arranged to ensure continued and optimal management of hypertension.

Severe BP elevation without any evidence of progressive target organ damage (*severe hypertension*) is often the result of inadequate treatment of pre-existing hypertension. These patients can be managed in an out-patient setting. Treatment should be aggressive in such patients with the concurrent use of two (or more) oral antihypertensive medications being a strong consideration. Achieving a significant reduction in BP within 48–72 h is a desired goal and will in most cases require a primary care provider for close follow-up and proper education. Emergency department physicians need to realize that severe elevations in BP alone may not represent an emergent situation. It is the clinical presentation as well as the presence of ongoing vascular target organ damage, not the degree of BP elevation itself, which dictates how emergent the circumstances are.

REFERENCES

1. Haas AR, Marik PE. Current diagnosis and management of hypertensive emergency. *Semin Dial* 2006; 19:502–512.
2. Monteiro FC Jr, Anunciação FA, Filho NS *et al.* Prevalence of true hypertensive crises and appropriateness of the medical management in patients with high blood pressure seen in a general emergency room. *Arq Bras Cardiol* 2008; 90:247–251.
3. Zampaglione B, Pascale C, Marchisio M *et al.* Hypertensive urgencies and emergencies: prevalence and clinical presentation. *Hypertension* 1996; 27:144–147.
4. Chobanian AV, Bakris GL, Black HR *et al.* Prevention, detection, evaluation, and treatment of high blood pressure. The JNC 7 Report. *JAMA* 2003; 289:2560–2571.

5. Elliot WJ. Clinical features and management of selected hypertensive emergencies. *J Clin Hypertens* 2004; 6:587–592.
6. Shayne PH, Pitts SR. Severely increased blood pressure in the emergency department. *Ann Emerg Med* 2003; 41:513–529.
7. Hebert CJ, Vidt DG. Hypertensive crises. *Prim Care Clin Office Pract* 2008; 35:475–487.
8. Moser M. Bed rest first for hypertensive emergencies? *J Clin Hyperetns (Greenwich)* 2008; 10:661.
9. Brooks TW, Finch CK, Lobo BL *et al*. Blood pressure management in acute hypertensive emergency. *Am J Health-Syst Pharm* 2007; 64:2579–2582.
10. Zeller KR, Von Kuhnert L, Mathews C. Rapid reduction of severe asymptomatic hypertension. A prospective, controlled trial. *Arch Intern Med* 1989; 149:2186.
11. Tisdale JE, Huang MB, Borzak S *et al*. Risk factors for hypertensive crisis: importance of out-patient blood pressure control. *Fam Pract* 2004; 21:420–424.
12. Tumlin JA, Dunbar LM, Oparil S *et al*. Fenoldopam, a dopamine agonist, for hypertensive emergency: a multicenter randomized trial: Fenoldopam Study Group. *Acad Emerg Med* 2000; 7:653–662.
13. Shea S, Misra D, Ehrlich MH *et al*. Predisposing factors for severe, uncontrolled hypertension in an inner-city minority population. *N Engl J Med* 1992; 327:776–778.
14. Vidt DG. Emergency room management of hypertensive urgencies and emergencies. *J Clin Hypertens (Greenwich)* 2001; 3:158–164.
15. Grossman E, Messerli FH. High blood pressure. A side effect of drugs, poisons, and food. *Arch Intern Med* 1995; 155:450–460.
16. Peters H, Baldwin M, Clarke M. The utility of laboratory data in the evaluation of the aysmptomatic hypertensive patient [abstract]. *Ann Emerg Med* 2002; 40:S48.
17. Rehman SU, Basile JN, Vidt D. Diagnosis and treatment of hypertensive crises. In: Black H, Elliott W (eds). *Clinical Hypertension: A Companion to Braunwald's Heart Disease*. Elsevier, Philadelphia, PA, 2007.
18. Kitiyakara C, Guzman NJ. Malignant hypertension and hypertensive emergencies. *J Am Soc Nephrol* 1998; 1046–6673/0901:133–142.
19. Grassi D, O'Flaherty M, Pellizzari M *et al*. Hypertensive urgencies in the ED: evaluating BP response to rest and to antihypertensive drugs with different profiles. *J Clin Hypertens (Greenwich)* 2008; 10:662–667.
20. Gifford RW. Management of hypertensive crises. *JAMA* 1991; 266:829–835.
21. Grossman E, Messerli FH, Grodzicki T *et al*. Should a moratorium be placed on sublingual nifedipine capsules given for hypertensive emergencies and pseudoemergencies? *JAMA* 1996; 276:1328–1331.
22. Jaker M, Atkin S, Soto M *et al*. Oral nifedipine vs oral clonidine in the treatment of urgent hypertension. *Arch Intern Med* 1989; 149:260–265.
23. White WB, Baker LH. Ambulatory blood pressure monitoring in patients with panic disorder. *Arch Intern Med* 1987; 147:1973–1975.
24. Gallagher EJ. Hypertensive urgencies: treating the mercury? *Ann Emerg Med* 2003; 41:530–531.
25. Marik PE, Varon J. Hypertensive crises: challenges and management. *Chest* 2007; 131:1949–1962.
26. Prisant LM, Carr AA, Hawkins DW. Treating hypertensive emergencies: controlled reduction of blood pressure and protection of target organs. *Postgrad Med* 1993; 93:92–110.
27. Strandgaard S, Paulson OB. Cerebral blood flow and its pathophysiology in hypertension. *Am J Hypertens* 1989; 2:486–492.
28. Vaughan CJ, Delanty N. Hypertensive emergencies. *Lancet* 2000; 356:411–417.
29. Cherney D, Strauss S. Management of patients with hypertensive urgencies and emergencies. A systematic review of the literature. *J Gen Intern Med* 2002; 19:937–945.
30. Perez MI, Musini VM. Pharmacological interventions for hypertensive emergencies. Cochrane Database of Systematic Reviews 2008, Issue 1. Art. No.: CD003653. DOI: 10.1002/14651858.CD003653.pub3.
31. Schwieler JH, Ericsson H, Löfdahl P, Thulin T, Kahan T. Circulatory effects and pharmacology of clevidipine, a novel ultra short acting and vascular selective calcium antagonist, in hypertensive humans. *J Cardiovasc Pharmacol* 1999; 34:268–274.
32. Nienaber CA, Eagle KA. Aortic dissection: new frontiers in diagnosis and management: Part II: therapeutic management and follow-up. *Circulation* 2003; 108:772–778.
33. Hamilton RJ, Carter WA, Gallagher EJ. Rapid improvement of acute pulmonary edema with sublingual captopril. *Acad Emerg Med* 1996; 3:205–212.

34. Francis GS, Siegel RM, Goldsmith SR *et al.* Acute vasoconstrictor response to intravenous furosemide in patients with chronic congestive heart failure. Activation of the neurohumoral axis. *Ann Intern Med* 1985; 103:1–6.

35. Sackner-Bernstein JD, Skopicki HA, Aaronson KD. Risk of worsening renal function with nesiritide in patients with acutely decompensated heart failure. *Circulation* 2005; 111:1487–1491.

36. Tietjen CS, Hurn PD, Ulatowski JA *et al.* Treatment modalities for hypertensive patients with intracranial pathology: options and risks. *Crit Care Med* 1996; 24:311–322.

37. Brott T, Lu M, Kothari R *et al.* Hypertension and its treatment in the NINDS rt-PA stroke trial. *Stroke* 1998; 29:1504–1509.

38. Adams HP Jr, del Zoppo G, Alberts MJ *et al.* Guidelines for the early management of adults with ischemic stroke. *Circulation* 2007; 15:e478–e534.

39. Broderick J, Connolly S, Feldmann E *et al*, American Heart Association; American Stroke Association Stroke Council; High Blood Pressure Research Council; Quality of Care and Outcomes in Research Interdisciplinary Working Group. Guidelines for the management of spontaneous intracerebral hemorrhage in adults: 2007 update: a guideline from the American Heart Association/American Stroke Association Stroke Council, High Blood Pressure Research Council, and the Quality of Care and Outcomes in Research Interdisciplinary Working Group. *Stroke* 2007; 38:2001–2023.

40. Mabie WC, Gonzalez AR, Sibai BM *et al.* A comparative trial of labetalol and hydralazine in the acute management of severe hypertension complicating pregnancy. *Obstet Gynecol* 1987; 70:328–333.

41. Frishman WH, Veresh M, Schlocker SJ, Tejani N. Pathophysiology and medical management of systemic hypertension in preeclampsia. *Curr Hypertens Rep* 2006; 8:502–511.

42. Hirschl MM, Binder M, Bur A *et al.* Safety and efficacy of Urapidil and sodium nitroprusside in the treatment of hypertensive emergencies. *Intensive Care Med* 1997; 23:885–888.

43. Wood A. Fenoldopam – a selective peripheral dopamine-receptor agonist for the treatment of severe hypertension. *N Engl J Med* 2001; 345:1548–1555.

44. Gonzales ER, Peterson MA, Racht EM *et al.* Dose response evaluation of oral labetalol in patients presenting to the emergency department with accelerated hypertension. *Ann Emerg Med* 1991; 20:333–338.

45. Singla N, Warltier DC, Gandhi SD *et al*, for the ESCAPE-2 Study Group. Treatment of acute postoperative hypertension in cardiac surgery patients: an Efficacy Study of Clevidipine Assessing Its Postoperative Antihypertensive Effect in Cardiac Surgery-2 (ESCAPE-2), a randomized, double-blind, placebo-controlled trial. *Anesth Analg* 2008; 107:59–67.

46. Levy JH, Mancao MY, Gitter R *et al.* Clevidipine effectively and rapidly controls blood pressure preoperatively in cardiac surgery patients: the results of the randomized, placebo-controlled Efficacy Study of Clevidipine Assessing its Pre-operative Antihypertensive Effect in Cardiac Surgery-1. *Anesth Analg* 2007; 105:918–925.

8

Managing hypertension in African American patients

J. M. Flack

BACKGROUND

Hypertension (HTN) in African Americans is a major clinical as well as public health problem. African Americans manifest an earlier onset, excess prevalence, and greater severity of hypertension compared to the white population. In addition, there is an excessively high burden of risk factors for hypertension in African Americans – obesity, physical inactivity, physiologically high level of dietary sodium intake, low levels of dietary potassium intake – that likely contribute to the high prevalence of hypertension in African Americans. Also, there is an inordinately high burden of pressure-related target organ injury in African Americans.

It has often been stated that hypertension in African Americans is the highest in the world. Well, this is partially true but not quite accurate. The age-adjusted prevalence rates of hypertension in adults residing in Spain, Finland, and Germany exceeds those in African Americans [1]. Thus, the prevalence of hypertension in African Americans is amongst the highest in the world but is not the highest.

Hypertension extracts an exceedingly high death toll from the African-American population. As many as 30% of all deaths in hypertensive African-American men and 20% in hypertensive African-American women are likely due to high blood pressure (BP). In 2005, the death rate from HTN (per 100 000 population) was 15.1 in white men, 51.0 in African-American men, 15.1 in white women and 40.9 in African-American women [2].

Pressure-related cardiovascular-renal complications – stroke, left ventricular hypertrophy (LVH), heart failure, chronic kidney disease (CKD)/end-stage renal disease (ESRD) – occur much more commonly in African Americans compared to whites [3]. This excess risk attributable to hypertension in African Americans relative to whites occurs for a multiplicity of reasons:

1. Earlier hypertension onset and thus longer duration of elevated BP.
2. Higher prevalence of severe (≥180/110 mmHg) BP elevations.
3. Lesser control of BP elevations.
4. A greater prevalence of risk enhancing morbidities such as diabetes and CKD.

John M. Flack, MD, MPH, FAHA, FACP, FACSG, Chairman, Department of Medicine; Chief, Division of Translational Research and Clinical Epidemiology, Wayne State University, Detroit Medical Center, Detroit, Michigan, USA.

The heterogeneity of risk factors for hypertension, hypertension incidence and prevalence, and therapeutic responses *within* the African-American population has received inadequate attention. This has, in no small part, been attributable to the pervasive notion that risk factors for hypertension, the burden of hypertension as well as therapeutic responses to various antihypertensive monotherapies, are reasonably similar amongst all African Americans. Nothing could be further from the truth. Accordingly, it has been well established that the prevalence of hypertension, as well as the prevalence of selected hypertension risk factors such as obesity, and also stroke risk, are higher amongst African Americans residing in the southeastern United States than amongst African Americans living elsewhere. One of the major contributors to an attenuated fall in BP response to commonly used antihypertensive drugs is high dietary sodium intake. Dietary sodium intake is much higher in less educated, lower income than higher educated, higher income African Americans. Interestingly, the prevalence of hypertension follows a similar trend.

Finally, lesser *average BP* responses to monotherapy with angiotensin converting enzyme (ACE) inhibitors and angiotensin receptor blockers (ARBs) in African Americans compared to whites has contributed significantly to the pervasive belief that African Americans do not respond to these agents. Nevertheless, as we have reported, the racial BP response distributions to these drugs overlap considerably and the largest variation in BP response, by far, is *within* each racial group not between them [4, 5]. A critical question that will be addressed later is the actual relevance of monotherapy drug responses to contemporary, optimal antihypertensive drug therapy.

WHAT PHENOTYPIC CHARACTERISTICS DISTINGUISH AFRICAN AMERICANS FROM WHITES WITH HYPERTENSION?

The short answer to this question is there are no phenotypic characteristics that reliably distinguish African American from white hypertensives. However, the subsequently described *group* differences do not reflect characteristics that are either present or absent in either racial group. Rather, each and every BP phenotypic difference subsequently described represents a qualitative not quantitative difference in BP/hypertension between African Americans and whites or any other race/ethnicity group.

Hypertension onset and severity

One of the most common differences is the prevalence of severe HTN ($\geq$180/100 mmHg), which is approximately 8-fold higher amongst African Americans than whites. Another phenotypic difference relates to the timing of hypertension onset. In African Americans the appearance of hypertension occurs earlier in life than has been observed amongst whites.

Diurnal ambulatory BP variation

The ambulatory BP phenotype differs, on average, in African Americans and whites. Normally night-time BP levels are 10–20% lower than daytime levels. African Americans, however, more often manifest 'non-dipping'. That is, the nocturnal ambulatory BP falls less than 10% from daytime levels. Nevertheless, more important than this observation of a racial difference in ambulatory BP phenotype is to understand the factors that vary at the individual level that are known to influence the diurnal variation in BP. Table 8.1 displays factors known to attenuate the nocturnal decline in BP. Several of these factors are related to diet and body habitus. Moreover, diurnal BP variation clearly responds to changes, for example, in diet. One of the more interesting observations has been that augmentation of dietary potassium intake to 80 mmol/day or higher, restores the normal nocturnal decline in BP in adolescent African-American females [6].

Table 8.1 Factors influencing the nocturnal decline in blood pressure.

Magnitude	
Greater	*Lesser*
■ Increased potassium intake ■ Nocturnal administration of: 　◆ Aspirin 　◆ Melatonin	■ Increased apnea-hypopnea ■ Evening/night shift work ■ Low socio-economic status ■ Male sex ■ Obesity ■ Post-menopausal ■ Increased sodium intake ■ Salt sensitivity ■ Increased sympathetic nervous system activity

Difficult-to-control hypertension

African-American hypertensives have been routinely characterized as a difficult to treat population subgroup. Hypertension control data from National Health and Nutrition Examination Survey (NHANES) III bears out that drug-treated African Americans with hypertension are less often controlled than their white counterparts [7]. It also appears that African Americans with hypertension manifest more of the individual characteristics/comorbidities – albuminuria, depressed kidney function, obesity, target organ injury, diabetes, and severe BP elevations – that have been linked to resistance to antihypertensive drug therapy and therefore lesser overall attainment of hypertension control [8, 9]. Over time, lesser attainment and maintenance of goal BP very likely contributes to the excessive risk of pressure-related complications in hypertensive African Americans.

Salt sensitivity

Salt sensitivity can be conceptualized by directionally appropriate BP changes occurring in response to increases or decreases in dietary sodium manipulations that exceed chance directionally appropriate random BP fluctuations. Assessing salt sensitivity in such a rigorous manner, however, is not feasible in clinical settings. Salt sensitivity, alternatively, has been diagnosed by directionally appropriate BP change after intravenous sodium loading or furosemide administration that exceeds an arbitrary threshold in mmHg. Salt sensitivity occurs in both normotensive as well as hypertensive persons of virtually all races. Some, though not all, studies have reported that salt sensitivity is more common in African American than white normotensives [10]. The racial disparity, however, has been more impressive amongst those with established hypertension [11]. Salt sensitivity is a modifiable, intermediate BP phenotype.

Again, the importance of the racial disparity in salt sensitivity pales in contrast to these questions. Firstly, what is the physiological and/or clinical relevance of salt sensitivity and secondly, what are the modifiable exposures that influence the BP response of the intact human to changes in dietary sodium?

Why does BP rise, at least in some individuals, when exposed to dietary sodium? One plausible explanation is that BP rises to enhance renal sodium excretion in an effort to maintain euvolemia. The higher BP is necessary to maintain steady state in/out sodium homeostasis, the major determinant of extracellular volume. The level of BP required to maintain steady state in/out sodium homeostasis can be influenced, for example, by nitric oxide deficiency and/or higher levels of angiotensin II, two factors that shift the pressure-

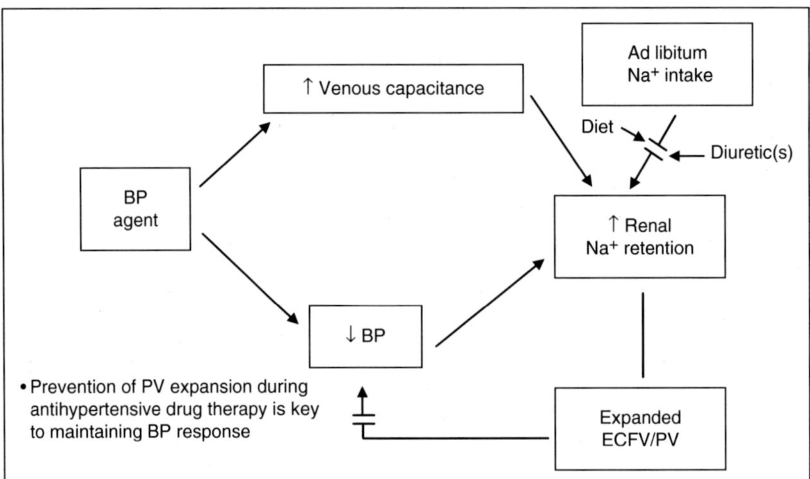

Figure 8.1 Expansion of extracellular fluid volume and attenuation of BP response. This figure displays a proposed mechanism through which antihypertensive drugs that expand venous capacitance (e.g. angiotensin converting enzyme inhibitors) induce salt sensitivity. These agents expand venous capacitance and therefore decentralize blood volume. In hypertensive (and obese) patients venous capacitance vessels are constricted. When BP falls and venous capacitance expands, and blood volume is decentralized, there is an augmentation of renal sodium excretion. Sodium retention continues until the vascular system is "full" again. This expansion of extracellular fluid volume/plasma volume (ECFV/PV) leads to diminution of the fall in BP unless the patient is given a diuretic and/or they restrict sodium intake to levels low enough to prevent plasma volume expansion.

natriuresis curve to the right. That is, a higher BP is needed to excrete the sodium load and to maintain euvolemia. In individuals or groups prone to salt sensitivity, the consumption of a typical western diet that contains sodium far in excess of physiological requirements, will likely lead to sustained BP elevations. Another reason for practitioners to be concerned about salt sensitivity is because salt sensitivity increases antihypertensive medication requirements and attenuates the fall in BP associated with many antihypertensive agents. We have put forth the hypothesis as displayed in Figure 8.1 that antihypertensive agents that not only lower BP but expand venous capacitance will decentralize blood volume and enhance renal sodium retention in an effort to "re-fill" the venous capacitance system. This will attenuate the fall in BP unless renal sodium reabsorption is prevented or attenuated by either dietary sodium restriction or concurrent diuretic therapy. In accordance with our hypothesis, antihypertensive drugs that appear especially prone to salt-induced attenuation of their BP lowering effect are renin-angiotensin system (RAS) blockers (e.g. ACE inhibitors), which are both arterial and venodilators; calcium antagonists, on the other hand, dilate the arterial but not the venous capacitance system. This likely explains the very modest attenuation of their BP lowering effect in the setting of high dietary sodium intake.

Suppressed circulating renin

African Americans have more often been shown to have suppressed circulating renin levels than whites. On the other hand, the majority of African Americans do not have suppressed circulating renin levels [12]. Nevertheless, this observation, along with lesser BP lowering with RAS blockers compared to either diuretics or calcium antagonists, has been the basis for the pervasive belief that the RAS system is less active in African Americans than whites. Nothing appears to be further from the truth.

A series of elegant studies has been interpreted to show that the local renal RAS system in healthy African Americans appears to be more active than in similar whites, and that there is incomplete suppression of the RAS after dietary sodium loading in African Americans [13, 14]. Furthermore, the pattern of pervasive pressure-related target organ injury in African Americans – excessive left ventricular hypertrophy, high rates of CKD – where the local RAS system is known to be overactive, is inconsistent with a quiescent RAS system in African Americans. Much of the underestimation of RAS activity in African Americans can also be traced to the erroneous and disproven notion, that activity of the circulating RAS system invariably corresponds to the activity of the predominate local RAS system.

WHICH PRESSURE-RELATED TARGET ORGAN INJURIES ARE MORE PREVALENT IN AFRICAN AMERICANS?

Vasculature

Both normotensive and hypertensive African Americans also manifest more endothelium-dependent and independent vascular dysfunction than whites. African Americans also have more micro- and macrovascular injury/remodeling, even at normotensive BP levels, than whites [15, 16].

Myocardium

African Americans have a higher prevalence of echocardiographic left ventricular hypertrophy than whites in many, though not all, studies of normotensives [17, 18], and also amongst hypertensives [19, 20]. Though this early myocardial adapation to pressure overload lowers wall stress, if maintained over the long term, there is a not inconsequential risk of developing heart failure. Thus, there should be little surprise that African Americans also have higher rates of heart failure than whites. Obesity is also a risk factor for heart failure and, especially amongst women, is more prevalent in African Americans than whites. Thus, excess obesity likely contributes to the excessive heart failure rates observed in African Americans.

Kidney

African Americans have approximately 4-fold higher rates of ESRD than their white counterparts [21]. Hypertension, *per se*, is a putative risk factor for CKD/ESRD. There is general acceptance of hypertension as a risk factor for CKD, although this paradigm is not universally accepted [22]. However, once CKD develops and renal function declines, the vast majority of individuals with CKD will manifest hypertension. And, BP control is important in patients with CKD, for not only the possible preservation of kidney function but also for the protection of other pressure-sensitive target organs.

Stroke

Stroke rates are several-fold higher in African Americans than whites. Stroke is a highly pressure-sensitive cardiovascular complication. Accordingly, the high rates of hypertension and lesser BP control over time in African Americans compared to whites undoubtedly has a major influence on the excess stroke risk in African Americans. Nevertheless, geographic residence importantly influences stroke risk in African Americans and to a lesser degree amongst whites. Stroke risk is approximately 50% greater amongst African Americans residing in the southeastern United States compared to those living elsewhere in the country.

WHICH ANTIHYPERTENSIVE DRUGS LOWER BLOOD PRESSURE MOST EFFECTIVELY IN AFRICAN AMERICANS WITH HYPERTENSION?

This question has long assumed great importance in determining the drugs recommended for African Americans with hypertension. Yet, it is at least arguable that this consideration is not very relevant in most African-American hypertensives. It has been well established that only a small minority of individuals of any race/ethnicity group achieve long-term BP control with a single antihypertensive agent. Even in clinical trials where African Americans were shown, on average, to respond better to diuretic and calcium antagonist monotherapy, the majority of them even taking these agents did not attain BP levels, on average, that were consistently below the most conservative contemporary JNC goal (<140/90 mmHg). In addition, as we have pointed out, the largest source of variation, by far, in response to angiotensin converting enzyme inhibitors, is within the racial groups not between them [4, 5]. Thus, the relevance of this question in regards to optimizing antihypertensive drug responses in African Americans must be viewed with jaded skepticism. Nevertheless, the most compelling reasons for the selection of antihypertensive drugs for an *individual* African-American hypertensive patient based on *group* BP responses would logically be the following:

1. To minimize the necessity of using more than one antihypertensive drug in individuals close to their goal BP (<15/10 mmHg); and/or
2. To lower BP with minimal cost in the absence of compelling indications for any given antihypertensive drug class, or contraindications to either a diuretic or calcium antagonist, preferential use of diuretics or generic calcium antagonists is very logical; these drug classes, on average, lower BP more than other drug classes in African Americans.

It should be explicitly stated that all antihypertensive drug classes lower BP effectively in African Americans. And, that the wide range of BP responses amongst African Americans to any drug class, irrespective of the average BP response for all African Americans, is too dissimilar to blanket extrapolate trends in average BP responses to all *individual* African Americans with hypertension. Drugs working primarily on the RAS – ACE inhibitors, ARBs, and β-blockers – have all been linked to lesser average BP responses than either diuretics or calcium antagonists in African Americans. However, when RAS blockers are combined with a diuretic or calcium antagonist, the BP lowering response is excellent and, for what it is worth, there is no racial differential in BP response. Thus, given the greater severity of hypertension as well as the excessive prevalence of comorbid conditions such diabetes, CKD and heart failure, there will be a need for the use of specific antihypertensive agents other than diuretics or calcium antagonists, irrespective of their magnitude of BP lowering.

The response to the acknowledgement of the tremendous variation in BP response in individuals of any racial group is to truly identify ways to individualize antihypertensive drug selection in a manner that matches individual characteristics in such a way that leads to greater BP lowering, enhanced target organ protection, and/or lesser risk of drug-related serious adverse consequences. Vascular phenotypic guidance of antihypertensive drug selection has, at least over the short term, proven useful in improving BP control rates both in primary care [23] and hypertension specialty practice [24] settings. The other obvious strategy is to identify gene polymorphisms that predict enhanced BP lowering, susceptibility to pressure-related complications, and/or increased risk to drug-related complications. Such approaches truly move antihypertensive treatment into the domain of personalized medicine. Blanket extrapolation of average group response to all *individuals* who comprise unknown positions in the spectrum of their group's response, though mistakenly labeled as individualization of therapy, is not. Old habits are hard to break. Nevertheless, in the ensuing years much more research and translation of these results needs to be done to satisfy the urgent need for guidance to practitioners on how to best treat their *individual* African-American patients with hypertension.

WHICH SOCIAL AND BEHAVIORAL FACTORS LIMIT ANTIHYPERTENSIVE THERAPEUTIC EFFECTIVENESS?

Successful long-term hypertension control represents the confluence of factors linked to the patient, the practitioner, the patient–provider interaction, and the system of care. As practitioners we routinely acknowledge very real, though sometimes perceived, patient shortcomings that lead to inadequate hypertension control. Non-compliance with antihypertensive medications is a common problem in the treatment of many chronic diseases. There are several potentially useful strategies that can affect compliance. However, virtually none of these strategies is optimally effective in isolation. Rather, they should be considered as most helpful when used in aggregate.

Psychobehavioral factors

Lesser hypertension control rates in African Americans do not appear to be attributable to taking hypertension less seriously as Bosworth and co-workers [25] reported that African Americans with hypertension actually perceived hypertension as a more serious condition than whites. However, African Americans were more likely to be non-adherent to prescribed therapeutic regimens as well as functionally illiterate. High levels of stress, worry about hypertension, experiencing antihypertensive medication side-effects, older age, and self-reporting medication non-adherence have all been linked to the African American excess in hypertension control [25–27].

Non-biomedical beliefs

African Americans with hypertension appear to manifest a significant number of non-biomedical beliefs that can interfere with long-term compliance with therapy and therefore serve to undermine hypertension control [28]. A significant number believe that hypertension can be cured or that hypertension medication should only be taken when experiencing symptoms. A surprising percentage believe that taking antihypertensive medication for life may not be necessary. Our experience has been that the number of antihypertensive medications is a significant emotional barrier to overcome. We repeatedly have to counsel patients regarding the fact that they are not "sicker" when taking four medications with controlled hypertension compared to when they were taking three medications with inadequately controlled hypertension. Yet, a surprising number of patients believe this to be the case. Even medications with higher milligram doses (240 mg vs. 4 mg) conjure up beliefs that they must be sicker if they are taking the more potent 240 mg tablet than the 4 mg tablet. Moreover, African Americans, as a group, tend to distrust the medical system more than their white counterparts.

Dietary sodium

The major dietary barrier to hypertension control has to do with excessive dietary sodium intake. Antihypertensive drugs that expand venous capacitance likely confer even greater salt sensitivity than is experienced by the same individual prior to being treated. There are several major hurdles to lowering dietary sodium intake. One is that dietary sodium enhances the taste of food and when it is removed food, at least initially, tastes blander. Another problem is that the sodium is mostly processed into the food before it is consumed or even cooked. Also, many patients erroneously believe that to effectively lower their dietary sodium intake all they have to do is to avoid adding sodium either during food preparation or at the table. It is also very difficult to control dietary sodium intake to reasonable levels (<2 g/day) when a significant number of meals are consumed outside of the home. Dietary sodium intake in African Americans also appears to be higher amongst those with less education and income [29].

Practitioner attitudes and patient–provider interactions

In African Americans there is a significant relationship between physician self-reported cultural competence and patient satisfaction as well as in their willingness to seek and share information during the medical visit [30]. African-American patients cared for by African-American physicians were more likely than those receiving care from non-African-American physicians to rate their physicians highly as well as to perceive that they received all needed medical care during the prior year [31]. Race concordance of the patient and physician appears to impact the clinic visit and patient perceptions of the clinic visit. Race-concordant clinic visits were longer, had higher ratings of positive patient affect, and were described as more participatory and more satisfying by patients [32].

Financial limitations

African Americans make less money, even with similar levels of education than whites, and also typically have less education as well. The lack of insurance coverage for a broad range of drugs limits practitioner options. However, by no means should potent, reasonably well-tolerated antihypertensive drug regimens be out of the reach of patients with financial constraints. Several of the large-chain pharmacies have hundreds of drugs offered for $4 per month. Included are thiazide diuretics, spironolactone, calcium antagonists, ACE inhibitors, reserpine, and β-blockers. Thus, it is possible to assemble a highly effective, four drug regimen for less than $20 per month.

SUMMARY

Inadequate hypertension control remains a problem in virtually all hypertensive populations in the United States as well as in most around the world. The adverse consequences of hypertension in African Americans are likely attributable to a multiplicity of factors:

1. Excessive hypertension prevalence.
2. Disproportionate prevalence of severe (≥180/110 mmHg) hypertension.
3. Inadequate BP control.
4. The high frequency of comorbid conditions – diabetes, albuminuria, CKD, and pressure-related target organ injury – all of which conspire to substantively amplify the risk of deleterious pressure-related outcomes, in part, because all confer resistance to the BP lowering effect of antihypertensive drug therapy.

After the diagnosis of hypertension has been conclusively made, all patients should undergo risk stratification, and after evaluating these risk factors, the goal BP level can be determined. There are several physiologic and non-physiologic factors that should be addressed in each individual patient to attain adequate BP control. There is no justification, at least in the minds of these authors, that black race, *per se*, justifies uniformly lower BP targets or avoidance of any particular class of antihypertensive agents such as those working primarily on the renin-angiotensin system. Rather we encourage appropriate risk stratification of all hypertensive patients.

REFERENCES

1. Cooper R, Rotimi C, Ataman S *et al.* The prevalence of hypertension in seven populations of west African origin. *Am J Public Health* 1997; 87:160–168.
2. National Center for Health Statistics, http://wonder.cdc.gov/mortSQL.html, 2008.
3. Burt V, Whelton P, Roccella E *et al.* Prevalence of hypertension in the US adult population. Results from the Third National Health and Nutrition Examination Survey, 1988–1991. *Hypertension* 1995; 25:305–313.
4. Mokwe E, Ohmit SE, Nasser SA *et al.* Determinants of blood pressure response to quinapril in black and white hypertensive patients: the Quinapril Titration Interval Management Evaluation trial. *Hypertension* 2004; 43:1202–1207.
5. Sehgal AR. Overlap between whites and blacks in response to antihypertensive drugs. *Hypertension* 2004; 43:566–572.
6. Wilson DK, Sica DA, Devens M, Nicholson SC. The influence of potassium intake on dipper and nondipper blood pressure status in an African-American adolescent population. *Blood Press Monit* 1996; 1:447–455.
7. Cutler JA, Sorlie PD, Wolz M, Thom T, Fields LE, Roccella EJ. Trends in hypertension prevalence, awareness, treatment, and control rates in United States adults between 1988–1994 and 1999–2004. *Hypertension* 2008; 52:818–827.
8. Cushman WC, Ford CE, Cutler JA *et al.* ALLHAT Collaborative Research Group. Success and predictors of blood pressure control in diverse North American settings: the Antihypertensive and Lipid-Lowering Treatment to Prevent Heart Attack Trial (ALLHAT). *J Clin Hypertens (Greenwich)* 2002; 4:393–404.
9. Nasser SA, Lai Z, O'Connor S, Liu X, Flack JM. Does earlier attainment of blood pressure goal translate into fewer cardiovascular events? *Curr Hypertens Rep* 2008; 10:398–404.
10. Wright JT Jr, Rahman M, Scarpa A *et al.* Determinants of salt sensitivity in black and white normotensive and hypertensive women. *Hypertension* 2003; 42:1087–1092.
11. Rodríguez Castellanos FE. Salt-sensitive hypertension. *Arch Cardiol Mex* 2006; 762:S161–S163.
12. Chrysant SG, Danisa K, Kem DC, Dillard BL, Smith WJ, Frohlich ED. Racial differences in pressure, volume and renin interrelationships in essential hypertension. *Hypertension* 1979; 1:136–141.
13. Price DA, Fisher ND, Osei SY, Lansang MC, Hollenberg NK. Renal perfusion and function in healthy African Americans. *Kidney Int* 2001; 59:1037–1043.
14. Price DA, Fisher ND, Lansang MC, Stevanovic R, Williams GH, Hollenberg NK. Renal perfusion in blacks: alterations caused by insuppressibility of intrarenal renin with salt. *Hypertension* 2002; 40:186–189.
15. Arnett DK, Rautaharju P, Crow R *et al.* Black–white differences in electrocardiographic left ventricular mass and its association with blood pressure (the ARIC study). Atherosclerosis Risk in Communities. *Am J Cardiol* 1994; 74:247–252.
16. Heffernan KS, Jae SY, Wilund KR, Woods JA, Fernhall B. Racial differences in central blood pressure and vascular function in young men. *Am J Physiol Heart Circ Physiol* 2008; 295:H2380–H2387.
17. Kamath S, Markham D, Drazner MH. Increased prevalence of concentric left ventricular hypertrophy in African-Americans: will an epidemic of heart failure follow? *Heart Fail Rev* 2006; 11:271–277.
18. Xie X, Liu K, Stamler J *et al.* Ethnic differences in electrocardiographic left ventricular hypertrophy in young and middle-aged employed American men. *Am J Cardiol* 1994; 73:564–567.
19. Antikainen R, Grodzicki T, Palmer AJ *et al.* The determinants of left ventricular hypertrophy defined by Sokolow-Lyon criteria in untreated hypertensive patients. *J Hum Hypertens* 2003; 17:159–164.
20. Lee DK, Marantz PR, Devereux RB *et al.* Left ventricular hypertrophy in black and white hypertensives. Standard electrocardiographic criteria overestimate racial differences in prevalence. *JAMA* 1992; 267:3294–3299.
21. Flessner MF, Wyatt SB, Akylbekova EL *et al.* Prevalence and awareness of CKD among African Americans: the Jackson Heart Study. *Am J Kidney Dis* 2009; 53:238–247.
22. Culleton BF, Larson MG, Wilson PW *et al.* Cardiovascular disease and mortality in a community-based cohort with mild renal insufficiency. *Kidney Int* 1999; 56:2214–2219.
23. Smith RD, Levy P, Ferrario CM; Consideration of Noninvasive Hemodynamic Monitoring to Target Reduction of Blood Pressure Levels Study Group. Value of noninvasive hemodynamics to achieve blood pressure control in hypertensive subjects. *Hypertension* 2006; 47:771–777.

24. Taler SJ, Textor SC, Augustine JE. Resistant hypertension: comparing hemodynamic management to specialist care. *Hypertension* 2002; 39:982–988.

25. Bosworth HB, Dudley T, Olsen MK *et al.* Racial differences in blood pressure control: potential explanatory factors. *Am J Med* 2006; 119:70.e9–e15.

26. Bosworth HB, Powers B, Grubber JM *et al.* Racial differences in blood pressure control: potential explanatory factors. *J Gen Intern Med* 2008; 23:692–698.

27. Roberts CB, Vines AI, Kaufman JS, James SA. Cross-sectional association between perceived discrimination and hypertension in African-American men and women: the Pitt County Study. *Am J Epidemiol* 2008; 167:624–632.

28. Ogedegbe G, Mancuso CA, Allegrante JP. Expectations of blood pressure management in hypertensive African-American patients: a qualitative study. *J Natl Med Assoc* 2004; 96:442–449.

29. Jen KL, Brogan K, Washington OG, Flack JM, Artinian NT. Poor nutrient intake and high obese rate in an urban African American population with hypertension. *J Am Coll Nutr* 2007; 26:57–65.

30. Paez KA, Allen JK, Beach MC, Carson KA, Cooper LA. Physician cultural competence and patient ratings of the patient–physician relationship. *J Gen Intern Med* 2009; 24:495–498.

31. Saha S, Komaromy M, Koepsell TD, Bindman AB. Patient–physician racial concordance and the perceived quality and use of health care. *Arch Intern Med* 1999; 159:997–1004.

32. Cooper LA, Roter DL, Johnson RL, Ford DE, Steinwachs DM, Powe NR. Patient-centered communication, ratings of care, and concordance of patient and physician race. *Ann Intern Med* 2003; 139:907–915.

9

Diagnostic considerations when evaluating hypertension in adolescents and patients less than 25 years of age

W. B. Moskowitz

BACKGROUND

Hypertension in children and adolescents had been considered relatively uncommon, with about 1–2% having blood pressure (BP) persistently above the 95th percentile for age, sex and weight percentile. Various factors are known to influence onset of primary hypertension in young people. Family history of hypertension and obesity are well-established risk factors. However, with the epidemic of childhood obesity and other environmental factors, BP has increased as has the prevalence of hypertension in young people [1]. This increase reflects an epidemiologic shift from secondary hypertension (most often caused by renal disease) to primary hypertension as the main cause of hypertension in school age children and adolescents. After three consecutive screenings of 6790 adolescents in Houston, Texas, 15.7% of the sample population was found to be persistently pre-hypertensive and 3.2% had hypertension [2]. Of 1717 eighth-grade students from 12 predominantly minority schools in three states (Texas, California, and North Carolina) 23.9% had hypertension, 16.7% had borderline total cholesterol, 4.0% had high cholesterol, 13.3% had low high-density cholesterol, and 17.2% had high triglycerides [3]. A total of 19.8% of the participants were at risk of being overweight and 29% were overweight. Associations between overweight and both elevated lipid and BP levels suggest that adolescents overweight or at risk for overweight should be screened for elevated BP and hyperlipidemia.

The aggregation of dyslipidemia, hypertension, and glucose intolerance defines the metabolic syndrome in adults and predicts the development of type 2 diabetes and cardiovascular disease (CVD). Obesity and BP track from childhood into adulthood. Blood pressures measured in childhood have been linked to hypertension and the metabolic syndrome in adulthood [4]. To remain free of hypertension or the metabolic syndrome, with or without hypertension, childhood BPs should remain below the 50th percentile for age and gender. The relative risk of adult hypertension for children with repeated measurements of systolic BP exceeding criterion values was greater for 5- to 7-year-old children than for older children and adolescents. These findings suggest that prevention of adult hypertension should

William B. Moskowitz, MD, FAAP, FACC, FSCAI, Professor, Pediatrics and Internal Medicine; Chair, Pediatric Cardiology; Director, Pediatric Cardiac Catheterization Laboratory; Vice Chair, Department of Pediatrics, Children's Medical Center, Medical College of Virginia, Virginia Commonwealth Universit.

begin in early childhood and that prevention and intervention programs may be more effective in younger children rather than older children and adolescents.

A revised population definition consistent with the adult hypertension terminology was presented in the fourth report of the National High Blood Pressure Education Program Working Group [5]. The BP must be obtained on three separate occasions. If the systolic and diastolic BP falls into different categories, the BP is classified by the higher category. Normal BP is defined as a systolic and diastolic BP below the 90th percentile for gender, age and height percentile. Pre-hypertension is defined as BP values consistently above the 90th percentile for age, gender, height, and adolescents with BP values above 120/80 mmHg but below the threshold for hypertension. Stage 1 hypertension is defined as a BP from the 95th percentile to 5 mmHg above the 99th percentile and Stage 2 hypertension is a BP above the 99th percentile plus 5 mmHg.

Among adults with pre-hypertension as many as 10% per year develop hypertension. In adolescent subjects for whom serial single BP measurements were obtained at intervals of 2 years, 21% of adolescent boys and 13% of adolescent girls met the criteria for pre-hypertension [6]. Fourteen percent of boys and 12% of the girls had hypertension 2 years later, indicating that the rate of progression of pre-hypertension to hypertension was approximately 7%. A high body mass index (BMI) at initial presentation and increasing BMI during the follow-up period predicted sustained BP elevations. Because both BP level and hypertension prevalence increase with age, young individuals with pre-hypertension will tend to progress to hypertension. Identification of adolescents with pre-hypertension and aggressive institution of lifestyle changes (weight control, salt restriction, exercise, and tobacco use cessation) may delay the need for pharmacologic intervention or successfully treat pre-hypertension.

Birth weight for gestational age, an indicator of fetal growth, has emerged as an independent predictor of adult high BP [7]. The Bogalusa Heart Study evaluated 185 children in a biracial cohort with complete follow-up data on birth weights and early childhood and adolescent anthropometric and BP measures to see if the later ethnic/racial differences in BP between black and white adolescents could be accounted for by initial differences in intrauterine growth [8]. Birth weights were a mean 443 and 282 g lower in black boys and girls, respectively, than in whites (P <0.001). Blood pressures in adolescence were 3.4/1.9 and 1.7/0.6 mmHg higher, respectively, and tracked from early childhood. In regression analyses, birth weight accounted for the ethnic difference in adolescent BP, which was also independently predicted by adolescent height, adolescent BMI, and systolic BP at 4 to 5 years of age and inversely by growth from 0 to 4 to 5 years. These results suggest that efforts to improve intrauterine growth in black infants as well as to lessen weight gain in adolescence may significantly reduce the excess of high BP/hypertension in this ethnic group.

WHAT ARE THE CARDIAC AND RENAL COMPONENTS OF THE WORK-UP FOR AN ADOLESCENT WITH HYPERTENSION?

Cardiac causes of secondary hypertension

Coarctation of the aorta, a common congenital heart defect, continues to be under diagnosed in adolescence and young adulthood, despite its ease of detection on physical examination alone. Coarctation is almost twice as common in males, is associated with a bicuspid aortic valve in up to 85% of cases with variable degrees of aortic stenosis and insufficiency, and is seen in approximately 35% of females with Turner syndrome. The anatomic obstruction is usually distal to the left subclavian artery and may be discrete or a long segment in length. The obstruction leads to bilateral upper extremity hypertension (in 10%, the right subclavian artery arises aberrantly distal to the coarctation, with hypertensive BPs being detected only in the left arm). Individuals with coarctation repaired in infancy and childhood may present with residual or recurrent coarctation due to either incomplete removal (or angioplasty +/- stenting) of the coarctated segment, residual transverse arch hypoplasia, or scarring of the initial repair. Late diagnosis after early childhood has a significant incidence of persistent hypertension following intervention, whether surgical or percutaneous.

The physical findings diagnostic of coarctation of the aorta are upper extremity hypertension, diminished femoral pulses with a femoral-brachial timing delay when palpated simultaneously. Bilateral brachial and femoral pulses should always be palpated. A systolic ejection click followed by a systolic ejection murmur at the base is consistent with a bicuspid aortic valve. An early diastolic murmur suggests aortic insufficiency. A long systolic or continuous murmur is usually heard in the interscapular area posteriorly over the spine and represents the turbulent flow through the coarcted segment. In adolescent and young adults with undiagnosed coarctation, collateral arteries enlarge to decompress the increased pressures in the upper body vascular bed and to supply blood to the lower body segments. The presence of these vessels is marked by continuous arterial murmurs heard over large portions of the chest and back.

Noninvasive confirmation of the diagnosis is made by echocardiogram with Doppler interrogation. This modality will define the anatomy and hemodynamic consequences of the coarctation, the presence and significance of a bicuspid aortic valve (and other defects such as patent ductus arteriosis, mitral valve disease, subaortic stenosis), the structural state of the myocardium and the level of cardiac function. Magnetic resonance imaging (MRI) and magnetic resonance angiography (MRA) are also useful not only as diagnostic modalities but as tools to monitor the patient after surgical or percutaneous interventions. Head MRI/MRA is suggested as well after the diagnosis of coarctation is confirmed as 5–8% of these individuals will have aneurysms of the vessels making up the circle of Willis.

If coarctation is clinically suspected but not found, other diagnoses that should be considered include "mid-aortic syndrome" or abdominal coarctation seen in individuals with William's syndrome and neurofibromatosis. Additionally, individuals who as infants required an umbilical arterial catheter may present with upper extremity hypertension due to obstruction from vascular remodeling of the abdominal aorta after thrombosis years earlier. Abdominal MRI/MRA will be diagnostic in such cases.

CARDIAC CHANGES IN PRIMARY HYPERTENSION

It is recommended that all young individuals with hypertension be evaluated with echocardiography. These individuals may have had a period of BP elevation prior to diagnosis and adverse cardiovascular (CV) changes may already be present. Neither the severity of casual BP elevations nor the presence of abnormal ambulatory blood pressure monitoring (ABPM) results at initial diagnosis is predictive of left ventricular hypertrophy (LVH). Left ventricular hypertrophy is frequently found in adults with essential hypertension and is well established as an important risk factor for CVD including sudden cardiac death. Echocardiography studies have shown that myocardial involvement may occur early in young hypertensive individuals. Left ventricular mass (LVM) increases during growth and thus normal must be defined in the context of the prevailing body size.

Pediatric and adolescent studies have reported frequencies of LVH from 8% to 38% in hypertensive individuals. In a recent study of 129 patients with a mean age of 13.6±3.6 years (67% male, 46.5% white, 38% African American, and 15.5% Hispanic), the prevalence of LVH was 15.5% using adult criteria and 41.1% using pediatric criteria [9]. Increasing BMI was associated with a higher LVM index. Using either pediatric or adult criteria, LVH was associated with BMI ≥95th percentile for age and gender. LVH and concentric hypertrophy were identified most frequently in Hispanic individuals.

The Strong Heart Study (1940 Native American participants, 14–39 years of age, mean age 29 years) analyzed clinical characteristics, hemodynamic parameters and LV structure and function in young individuals [10]. Hypertension occurred in 15% and pre-hypertension in 35%. Both hypertensive and pre-hypertensive participants had higher LV wall thickness and LVM, and 3- and 2-fold higher prevalences respectively of LVH than their normotensive counterparts did. In another study, 67 consecutive children and adolescents (ages 5–16 years) characterized as hypertensive or pre-hypertensive using ambulatory blood pressure (ABP) criteria exhibited significantly higher LVM index than did normotensive individuals [11].

Young individuals with white coat hypertension were found to have LVM index values that fell between sex, age and BMI matched individuals with sustained hypertension and those who were normotensive [12]. In another study, 119 young people (mean age 13.3 years; 65% male) were evaluated for their hypertension [13]. Left ventricular mass index exceeded the 95th percentile for age/sex in 59% of males and 90% of females in the persistent hypertension group and in 33% of males and 36% of females in the white coat hypertension (WCH) group. These studies suggest that WCH may not be totally benign and may be associated with pressure-related end-organ effects in young people.

Finally, young individuals with persistent masked hypertension or who progressed to sustained mild hypertension over a 37-month median follow-up period had a higher LVM index and a higher percentage of LVM index values above the 95th percentile (30% versus 0%; P = 0.014) than did normotensive controls [14]. Masked hypertension is a likely precursor of sustained hypertension and LVH. Therefore, individuals diagnosed with sustained hypertension or lesser degrees of hypertension (pre-, masked-, or "white coat") should undergo a comprehensive echocardiographic evaluation as they may be at similar risk for target organ damage.

RENAL CAUSES OF SECONDARY HYPERTENSION

Renal disease and renal vascular disease are by far the commonest causes of secondary hypertension in young people, accounting for 80–90% of such patients.

Chronic renal disease

A history of recurrent urinary tract infections, congenital anatomic, renal, ureteral, or bladder abnormalities, genetic cystic disease (autosomal recessive polycyctic disease), or excessive use of analgesics or other nephrotoxic drugs should be sought. Chronic kidney disease (CKD), cystic renal disease or renal interstitial disease in hypertensive patients virtually always is associated with an abnormal urinalysis or laboratory evidence of renal insufficiency.

The presence of proteinuria is always of clinical concern because it indicates glomerular disease and albuminuria strongly predicts the risk of end-stage renal disease (ESRD) and cardiovascular (CV) risk. Patients with proteinuria (that is not of the orthostatic variant) should be screened for diabetes mellitus and connective tissue disease. Microalbuminuria is present in about 9% of adolescents [15]. The prevalence of microalbuminuria is higher among non-overweight than overweight adolescents. The median albumin/creatinine ratio decreases with increasing BMI z scores. Among overweight adolescents, microalbuminuria is associated with impaired fasting glucose, insulin resistance, hypertension, and smoking, as well as diabetes mellitus and not increasing BMI *per se*.

Renal insufficiency is most commonly recognized by measurement of serum creatinine values, which are more reliable than blood urea nitrogen (BUN), due to the influence of hydration status, dietary protein intake, and overall nutrition on the latter. Therefore, in addition to urinalysis (red blood cells and red cell casts are hallmark findings of glomerular disease), evaluation should include urine albumin:creatinine, serum creatinine, BUN, electrolytes, creatinine clearance, and a renal ultrasound. Renal ultrasonography is quite useful in defining renal size and symmetry, identifying cysts and aiding in the diagnosis of obstructive uropathy. Renal biopsy is reserved for situations where the information may contribute to treatment or patient prognosis.

Renal vascular hypertension

Renal vascular disease (renal artery stenosis) is the third most common pathologic condition (after renal scarring and glomerular disease) resulting in significant sustained hypertension in young people. Renal vascular disease is the cause of hypertension in 4% to 20% of children and adolescents with hypertension. Renal artery stenosis may be found in association with Turner's or Williams's syndromes, neurofibromatosis, or as a part of a more diffuse fibromuscular dysplasia syndrome involving the abdominal aorta and its major branches. Bilateral renal artery stenosis can be seen in almost half the patients and intrarenal disease occurs in 45% of patients [16]. It is recommended that routine cerebrovascular imaging be performed on all children and young adults with renal artery stenosis, because it is not possible to predict cerebrovascular disease (seen in 25–30% of patients) based on the nature or extent of renal vascular involvement alone. The presence of an abdominal bruit or posterior flank bruit (auscultation in a quiet room, with patient supine) suggests renal artery stenosis.

Non-invasive imaging studies are typically used for initial diagnosis. In association with renal ultrasound studies, Doppler interrogation of the renal arteries can produce reliable estimates of renal blood flow and gradients across stenotic vessels. Dynamic imaging using high-speed CT can provide measurements of parenchymal volume and perfusion, but do utilize iodinated contrast agents, an increased risk for patients with renal insufficiency. Magnetic resonance angiography with gadolinium can visualize the major renal arteries and renal architecture, assess the degree of stenosis, and estimate renal function by measuring clearance of the contrast agent. Its value is limited on gaining insight into the structure of more distal or accessory vessels.

To identify lesions potentially remediable with angioplasty or stenting techniques, patients can undergo pre-captopril (or any other ACE inhibitor) and post-captopril scintigraphy with dimercaptosuccunic acid (DMSA) labeled with technetium-99m and selective renal vein renin sampling with segmental sampling. Intra-arterial DSA with renal venous renin measurements has been shown to be an accurate method of diagnosing renal vascular hypertension. It may be used as an initial screening examination in patients with suspected renal vascular hypertension as well as a useful technique for interventional vascular procedures and follow-up. Conventional angiography of the aorta and renal arteries is now most commonly performed at the time of planned endovascular intervention or prior to surgical therapy.

WHAT IS THE ROLE OF 24-H AMBULATORY BLOOD PRESSURE MONITORING AND HOME BLOOD PRESSURE MONITORING IN THE ADOLESCENT WITH HYPERTENSION?

A recent study of 118 patients (aged 3–19 years) with CKD compared ABPM, self-measurement of BP at home, and clinic BP measurements [17]. Self-measured BP was shown to be a valuable addition to clinic BP measurement, as it agreed with ABPM more closely and more consistently over the range of BP compared with clinic BP alone. However, the diagnostic sensitivity reached by self-measured BP and clinic BP was only 81% compared with ABPM as the reference method. Therefore, 1 of 5 children diagnosed as hypertensive by ABPM would have been missed, even when both clinic BP and self-measured BP were used in combination.

ABPM has gained acceptance as a useful modality for the evaluation of BP levels in young people. A recent scientific statement from the American Heart Association summarizes the current research and clinical applications of ABPM in young people and offers recommendations on implementation of ABPM in practice and interpretation of results [18]. Indications where ABPM may prove useful are given in Table 9.1.

Ambulatory blood pressure monitoring has been used to help differentiate secondary hypertension from primary hypertension in young people. Ninety-seven ABPM studies were obtained from 85 individuals (aged 13.8±3.5 years) 40 of whom had primary hyperten-

Table 9.1 The indications for ambulatory BP monitoring.

<table>
<tr><td>

1 Confirming the diagnosis of hypertension
  a. To determine presence of true hypertension or WCH
  b. To evaluate for the presence of masked hypertension when there is clinical suspicion of
    hypertension but normal casual hypertension
  c. To evaluate the effects of medications used for comorbid conditions (e.g. ADHD)
2 Assessing BP variability
  a. To determine dipping status in patients at high risk for end-organ damage
  b. To assess the severity and persistence of BP elevation
3 Evaluating the effectiveness of drug therapy for hypertension
  a. To evaluate apparent drug-resistant hypertension
  b. To determine whether symptoms can be attributed to drug-related hypotension
4 Evaluating BP levels more accurately in chronic pediatric diseases associated with hypertension

</td></tr>
<tr><td>

ADHD = attention deficit hyperactivity disorder; BP = blood pressure; WCH = white coat hypertension.

</td></tr>
</table>

sion and 57 who had secondary hypertension [19]. Daytime diastolic and nocturnal systolic BP loads were significantly greater in patients with secondary hypertension. A daytime diastolic BP load of ≥25% and/or a nocturnal systolic BP load of ≥50% was highly specific for secondary hypertension. In another study, ABPM studies were analyzed from 145 young people with untreated hypertension; 45 had primary hypertension while 100 had secondary hypertension [20]. Subjects with secondary hypertension had a lesser nocturnal BP dip for systolic and diastolic BP in comparison to those with primary hypertension. Eleven percent of those with primary hypertension were classified as non-dippers (BP dip >10%) for systolic BP and no one was a non-dipper for diastolic BP; alternatively, of those with secondary hypertension, 65% were nondippers for systolic and 21% for diastolic BP. Nocturnal systolic and diastolic BP loads were significantly greater in those with secondary hypertension.

Obese adolescents have higher ambulatory BP readings and greater carotid artery intimal-medial thickness (CIMT) than those who were not obese [21]. Mean 24-h, daytime, and night-time systolic BP were significantly higher in obese subjects compared with non-obese subjects (P <0.002), the magnitude of systolic white coat effect was significantly higher in obese subjects (P <0.006) and WCH was significantly more frequent in obese subjects (P <0.0001). These studies demonstrate that arterial wall changes may already be present in young obese hypertensives. In the face of the evolving epidemic in children and young adults of obesity, hypertension, type 2 diabetes mellitus, and dyslipidemia, the use of ABPM is likely to increase as a means to define present and future CV risk. Interestingly, in obese pre-pubertal children with substantial weight loss resulting from participation in a 1-year outpatient intervention program, CIMT, BP, triglycerides, insulin, and insulin resistance index decreased significantly, whereas high-density lipoprotein cholesterol increased significantly [22]. Paralleling the improvement of the CV risk factor profile with substantial weight loss, CIMT also decreased in obese children, suggesting some degree of reversibility to these early atherosclerotic changes.

Impairment of nocturnal BP regulation has been consistently reported in adolescents and young adults with type 1 diabetes mellitus [23]. Ambulatory blood pressure monitoring was performed in 2105 children and adolescents with type 1 diabetes mellitus. Nocturnal BP in particular was significantly elevated and dipping of SBP, DBP, and MAP was significantly reduced (P <0.0001). Age, diabetes duration, sex, BMI, hemoglobin A_1C, and insulin dose were related to altered BP profiles; dipping, however, was affected by age, female sex, and hemoglobin A_1C. The presence of microalbuminuria was associated with nocturnal DBP (P <0.0001) and degree to which DBP dipped (P <0.01).

WHAT IS THE ROLE OF PSYCHIATRIC COMORBIDITIES AND ANY ASSOCIATED THERAPIES IN THE ADOLESCENT WITH HYPERTENSION AND A PSYCHIATRIC DISORDER?

Adolescence is often characterized as a rebellious, emotionally labile, tumultuous period of development. Behavioral responses are learned within the constraints of gender-role socialization, which may cause adolescent boys and girls to respond to angering stimuli differently. The relationship of emotions and emotional behavioral factors to the development of hypertension was evaluated in 63 urban high school seniors aged 16–18 years [24]. Hypertension was noted in 43% of the total sample with 65% of boys and 27% of girls having BP readings ≥95th percentile. Another 10% were found to be pre-hypertensive. Both systolic and diastolic BP increased with BMI for both genders. Analysis revealed significant positive relationships between anger expression with BP, and a significant inverse relationship between BP and the control of anger for girls. Girls scored higher on levels of overall anger and anger-out than the boys, with both of these patterns of anger expression being significantly related to BP. Mismanaged anger is therefore a potentially modifiable risk factor in adolescence, and specific interventions can be focused on modifying the ineffective expression of anger to promote improved overall health.

Psychiatric comorbidity has been detected in adolescents, especially those with oppositional defiance, anxiety, and attention deficit hyperactivity disorder (ADHD). Use of stimulant medications, which also increase CV reactivity, results in higher heart rates and ambulatory BP values in children with ADHD [25]. In a double-blind, randomized, cross-over trial, a significantly higher ABPM rate pressure product was found in children receiving active treatment for ADHD. Elevated rate pressure product is an index of myocardial oxygen demand, suggesting that stimulant medications may significantly increase metabolic demands on the CV systems of children being treated for ADHD. Blood pressure and heart rate screening and monitoring during stimulant therapy to determine whether alterations become clinically significant is advisable.

While 7–12% of youth are estimated to be affected with ADHD, longitudinal data coupled with survey and epidemiological studies suggest that 4% of adults in the general population manifest ADHD. Compared to non-ADHD adults, controlled studies indicate that adults with ADHD have higher rates of comorbid psychopathology, occupational and/or academic underachievement, and interpersonal difficulties necessitating treatment [26]. In a recent study of 125 adult subjects with ADHD (aged 39±9 years), both stimulant and nonstimulant catecholaminergic medications were associated with minor but statistically significant changes in heart rate and BP [27]. New onset cases of systolic or diastolic hypertension (BP ≥140/90 mmHg) were recorded in 8% of placebo-treated subjects and 10% of subjects receiving active medication, regardless of the class of medication. Given the minor pressor and chronotropic effect of these medications, adult patients with ADHD should have BP (and heart rate patterns) evaluated at baseline and periodically during therapy.

Poor adherence to antihypertensive medications is common and negatively impacts CV morbidity risk. Adverse drug effects contribute to this problem. However, some patients who repeatedly discontinue medications may misinterpret non-specific symptoms as drug side-effects, because of a psychiatric disorder. Hypertension is significantly associated with panic disorder, anxiety, and panic attacks, which may mimic adverse drug reactions [28]. A survey of hypertensive patients with two or more drug intolerances found significant associations with panic attacks ($P = 0.008$), anxiety ($P = 0.02$), and depression ($P = 0.02$) [29]. In that study of 276 patients, the blood pressure was higher by an average of 8/4 mmHg in patients who had previously experienced two or more episodes of nonspecific drug intolerance, and 15/16 mmHg in patients who had experienced five or more non-specific episodes. Thus, multiple-drug intolerance was associated with inadequate blood pressure control. Panic disorder, which is far more commonly diagnosed after the diagnosis of hypertension than before, does tend to make treatment of hypertension more difficult. Recognition and treatment of underlying psychiatric comorbidities may lead to more successful implementation of antihypertensive therapy.

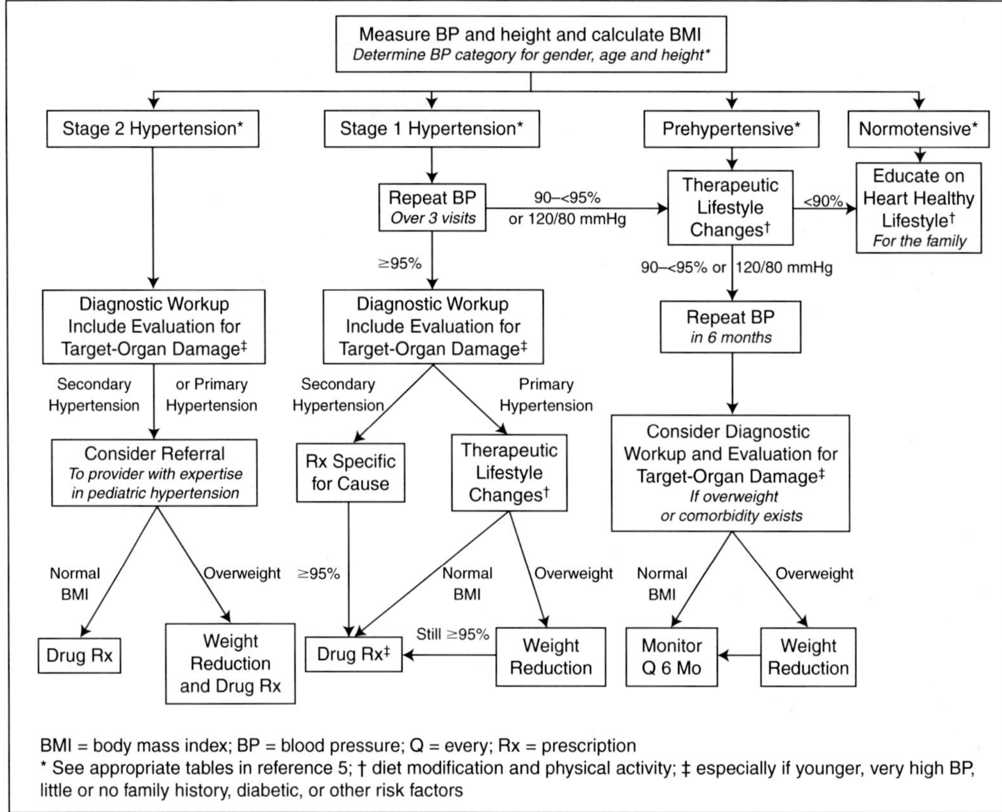

Figure 9.1 Treatment algorithm for hypertension in young people (with permission from [5]).

Various psychiatric disorders are associated with an increased prevalence of CV disease. Cardiovascular mortality in schizophrenia exceeds that of the general population. The management of chronic medical conditions such as hypertension requires the patient to accomplish a series of tasks, including engaging in healthful activities, monitoring physical symptoms, and signs, and interacting with healthcare providers. A cross-sectional study evaluated the interrelationships of psychiatric symptom severity, medical comorbidity, and psychosocial functioning from 50 sites in the US [30]. Of the 1424 participants in the study sample (aged 40.6±11.1 years), 58% had at least one medical condition: 20% had hypertension, 11% diabetes mellitus, and 9% had four or more medical conditions. Medical comorbidities were associated with poorer neurocognitive functioning and greater depressive symptoms. Therefore, not only may medical conditions and their therapies cause additional cognitive impairment, but cognitive impairment may also lead to exacerbations of comorbidities seen in patients with psychiatric disorders.

ARE THERE ANY PREFERRED THERAPIES IN THE TREATMENT OF HYPERTENSION IN THE ADOLESCENT AND WHAT IS A GOAL BLOOD PRESSURE?

The fourth report of the National High Blood Pressure Education Program (NHBPEP) describes the approach to treatment of hypertension in young people [5]. The treatment algorithm takes into account the severity of BP elevation, the likelihood of secondary hypertension, the presence of target organ involvement such as LVH, and the presence of comorbidities such as obesity, diabetes mellitus, and renal disease (Figure 9.1). Because of the growing obesity epidemic in young people, screening for dyslipidemia and glucose intolerance and counseling about tobacco consumption must be incorporated into the management of hypertension.

Therapeutic lifestyle changes are currently recommended as the initial approach for young people with less severe hypertension or those with primary hypertension and no target organ involvement. For those hypertensive individuals who are overweight or obese, dietary modification, physical activity, and behavioral therapy are useful to manage weight. These interventions should be the mainstay of therapy in young people with hypertension, even if pharmacologic therapy is required.

Adolescent obesity is a major public health problem. Despite widespread and long-standing appreciation of the importance of diet and exercise to reduce overweight and obesity, the evidence suggests that weight-loss programs for adolescents are only modestly successful. However, a comprehensive lifestyle modification program used in adults aged 25 years and older demonstrated in a randomized clinical trial that individuals with pre-hypertension and stage 1 hypertension can make and sustain lifestyle changes resulting in improved hypertension control and reduced CV risk [31].

The serotonin and norepinephrine reuptake inhibitor sibutramine is approved for the management of adult obesity. The results of a 12-month, randomized, double-blind, placebo-controlled study that evaluated the efficacy and safety of sibutramine in addition to behavioral therapy in obese adolescents 12–16 years of age with multiethnic backgrounds and BMIs of 28.1 to 46.3 kg/m^2 were recently published [32]. At the endpoint, there was a mean treatment group difference in BMI of 2.6 kg/m^2 in favor of sibutramine. Small mean decreases in BP and pulse rate were seen in both sibutramine and placebo groups. Reductions in vital signs were greater when BMI reduction was ≥5% compared with <5%. The odds ratio for achieving ≥5% BMI reduction with sibutramine treatment compared to placebo was 10.1 (P <0.001). In a young, growing population, even small losses in BMI or even maintenance of BMI are important outcomes that will influence related comorbidities. The use of sibutramine treatment in obese hypertensive adolescents in addition to diet, exercise, and behavioral therapy may promote weight loss with concomitant improvement in BP.

Indications for initiating pharmacologic therapy include:

1. Symptomatic hypertension.
2. Secondary hypertension.
3. Evidence of target organ damage.
4. Diabetes mellitus (types 1 and 2).
5. Persistent hypertension despite non-pharmacologic measures [33].

Existing causes of secondary hypertension such as renal, cardiac, or endocrine diseases often mandate the choice of initial pharmacologic agent. Drugs acting on the renin-angiotensin system, such as angiotensin converting enzyme (ACE) inhibitors and angiotensin-receptor blockers are preferred in patients with renal disease, as they slow the progression of renal failure as well as reduce proteinuria.

Persistent hypertension following adequate correction of coarctation of the aorta without a significant residual gradient is initially treated with a β-blocker, though ACE inhibitors may also be used with the added benefit of promoting myocardial remodeling. As in adults, hypertensive adolescents with either type 1 or 2 diabetes mellitus should be treated with an ACE inhibitor or an angiotensin-receptor blocker (ARB), as these agents are known to slow if not, in certain cases, prevent the development of diabetic nephropathy.

The goals of therapy are defined in the NHBPEP report [5]. Individuals with uncomplicated primary hypertension and no evidence of target organ damage should have a goal for

BP reduction to <95th percentile for age, sex, and height. For individuals with secondary hypertension, diabetes mellitus, or hypertensive target organ damage, the BP goal is <90th percentile for age, sex, and height.

All classes of hypertensive agents appear to be effective in reducing BP in young people. The results of a survey of North American pediatric nephrologists showed that the most commonly used first line agent with primary hypertension were ACE inhibitors 46.7% and calcium-channel blockers (CCBs) 36.8% [34]. Diuretics were used by 15.3% and β-blockers by 6.6%. Second line agents were CCBs 39%, and ACE inhibitors, 32.9%. Diuretics were used as a second line agent in 13.7% and β-blockers by 17%. Angiotensin receptor blockers were used as a second line agent in 4.9%.

The goal BP of therapy is not achieved in a significant percentage of patients. A major reason for this is lack of patient adherence to non-pharmacologic as well as pharmacologic therapies. Factors that affect adherence to treatment include, among others, the complexity of the regimen and the side-effects of medication used [35]. Therefore, long-acting agents given once daily, agents with few adverse effects, and fixed dose combinations may offer the best chance for patient compliance. Escalating the dose of a medication every six weeks appears to provide optimal BP control with fewer adverse effects.

SUMMARY

Chronic hypertension is becoming increasingly common in adolescence and young adulthood. While causes of secondary hypertension should always be sought, especially in younger children, primary hypertension predominates in young adults and is generally associated with obesity, sedentary lifestyle, and a positive family history of hypertension and other cardiovascular risk factors. Young individuals with hypertension, even mild hypertension may have end organ damage due to elevated BP for a period of time before diagnosis. Therefore, young individuals diagnosed with sustained hypertension or lesser degrees of hypertension (pre-, masked-, or white coat hypertension) should undergo a comprehensive echocardiographic evaluation as they may be at similar risk for target organ damage. Ambulatory blood pressure monitoring is a useful modality in diagnosing the presence of and type of hypertension as well as monitoring the effects of lifestyle modification and efficacy of pharmacologic therapy.

Atherosclerosis begins in childhood and progresses during adolescence and young adulthood [36]. A fasting lipid profile is recommended in all overweight patients with pre-hypertension and in all hypertensive patients, as well as those with a family history of dyslipidemia, hypertension, or premature atherosclerosis. The best approach to prevention of future CV disease in these young individuals is early recognition and aggressive therapy. The indications for pharmacologic therapy include symptomatic hypertension, secondary hypertension, an insufficient response to lifestyle modification, or the presence of target organ involvement. The goal of therapy should be BP reduction below the 95th percentile unless concurrent conditions are present; in those situations, BP should be reduced to below the 90th percentile. Poor adherence to antihypertensive medications is common in this age group. While drug side-effects may contribute to this problem, some patients who repeatedly discontinue medications may misinterpret non-specific symptoms as drug side-effects, because of a comorbid psychiatric disorder. Prevention of adult hypertension should begin in early childhood. Prevention and intervention programs are likely more effective in younger children rather than older children, adolescents, or young adults.

REFERENCES

1. Muntner P, He J, Cutler JA *et al.* Trends in blood pressure among children and adolescents. *JAMA* 2004; 291:2107–2113.

2. McNeice KL, Poffenbarger TS, Turner JL *et al.* Prevalence of hypertension and pre-hypertension among adolescents. *J Pediatr* 2007; 150:640–644.

3. Jago R, Harrell JS, McMurray RG *et al.* Prevalence of abnormal lipid and blood pressure values among an ethnically diverse population of eighth-grade adolescents and screening implications. *Pediatrics* 2006; 117:2065–2073.

4. Sun SS, Grave GD, Siervogel RM *et al.* Systolic blood pressure in childhood predicts hypertension and metabolic syndrome later in life. *Pediatrics* 2007; 119:237–247.

5. National High Blood Pressure Education Program Working Group on High Blood Pressure in Children and Adolescents. The fourth report on the diagnosis, evaluation, and treatment of high blood pressure in children and adolescents. *Pediatrics* 2004; 114:555–576.

6. Falkner B, Gidding SS, Portman R *et al.* Blood pressure variability and classification of prehypertension and hypertension in adolescence. *Pediatrics* 2008; 122:238–242.

7. Huxley RR, Shiell AW, Law CM. The role of size at birth and postnatal catch-up growth in determining systolic blood pressure. *J Hypertens* 2000; 18:815–831.

8. Cruickshank JK, Mzayek F, Liu L *et al.* Origins of the "black/white" difference in blood pressure. Roles of birth weight, postnatal growth, early blood pressure, and adolescent body size. The Bogalusa Heart Study. *Circulation* 2005; 111:1932–1937.

9. Hanevold C, Waller, Daniels S *et al.* The effects of obesity, gender, and ethnic group on left ventricular hypertrophy and geometry in hypertensive children: a collaborative study of the International Pediatric Hypertension Association. *Pediatrics* 2004; 113:328–333.

10. Drukeinis JS, Roman MJ, Fabsitz RR *et al.* Cardiac and systemic hemodynamic characteristics of hypertension and prehypertension in adolescents and young adults: the Strong Heart Study. *Circulation* 2007; 115:221–227.

11. Stabouli S, Kotsis V, Karagianni C *et al.* Left-ventricular mass index in hypertensive children and adolescents. *Pediatrics* 2008; 121:S96.

12. Lande MB, Meagher CC, Gross Fisher S *et al.* Left ventricular mass index in children with white coat hypertension. *J Pediatr* 2008; 153:50–54.

13. Kavey RW, Kveselis DA, Ataliah N *et al.* White coat hypertension in childhood: evidence for end-organ effect. *J Pediatr* 2007; 150:491–497.

14. Lurbe E, Torro I, Alvarez V *et al.* Prevalence, persistence, and clinical significance of masked hypertension in youth. *Hypertension* 2005; 45:493–498.

15. Nguyen S, McCulloch C, Brakeman P *et al.* Being overweight modifies the association between cardiovascular risk factors and microalbuminuria in adolescents. *Pediatrics* 2008; 121:37–45.

16. Shroff R, Roebuck DJ, Gordon I *et al.* Angioplasty for renovascular hypertension in children: 20-year experience. *Pediatrics* 2006; 118:268–275.

17. Wuhl E, Hadtstein C, Mehls O *et al.* Home, clinic, and ambulatory blood pressure monitoring in children with chronic renal failure. *Pediatr Res* 2004; 7:21–25.

18. Urbina E, Alpert B, Flynn J *et al.* Ambulatory blood pressure monitoring in children and adolescents: recommendations for standard assessment. A scientific statement from the American Heart Association Atherosclerosis, Hypertension, and Obesity in Youth Committee of the Council on Cardiovascular Disease in the Young and the Council for High Blood Pressure Research. *Hypertension* 2008; 52:433–451.

19. Flynn JT. Differentiation between primary and secondary hypertension in children using ambulatory blood pressure monitoring. *Pediatrics* 2002; 110:89–93.

20. Seeman T, Palyzova D, Dusek J *et al.* Reduced nocturnal blood pressure dip and sustained nighttime hypertension are specific markers of secondary hypertension. *J Pediatr* 2005; 147:366–371.

21. Stabouli S, Kotsis V, Papamichael C *et al.* Adolescent obesity is associated with high ambulatory blood pressure and increased intimal-medial thickness. *J Pediatr* 2005; 147:651–656.

22. Wunsch RW, de Sousa G, Toschke AM *et al.* Intima-medial thickness in obese children before and after weight loss. *Pediatrics* 2006; 118:2334–2340.

23. Dost A, Klinkert C, Kapellen T *et al.* Arterial hypertension determined by ambulatory blood pressure profiles. *Diabetes Care* 2008; 31:720–725.

24. Starner TM, Peters RM. Anger expression and blood pressure in adolescents. *J Sch Nurs* 2004; 20:335–342.

25. Samuels JA, Franco K, Wan F *et al.* Effect of stimulants on 24-h ambulatory blood pressure in children with ADHD: a double-blind, randomized, cross-over trial. *Pediatr Nephrol* 2006; 21:92–95.

26. Wilens T, Spencer T, Biederman J. A review of the pharmacotherapy of adults with attention-deficit/ hyperactivity disorder. *J Atten Disord* 2002; 5:189–202.

27. Wilens TE, Hammerness PG, Biederman J *et al*. Blood pressure changes associated with medication treatment of adults with attention-deficit/hyperactivity disorder. *J Clin Psychiatry* 2005; 66:253–259.

28. Handler J. Refractory hypertension: recognition of psychiatric comorbidity. *J Clin Hyperten* 2003; 5:235–236.

29. Davies SJ,Jackson PR, Ramsay LE *et al*. Drug intolerance due to nonspecific morbidity in hypertension patients. *Arch Intern Med* 2003; 163:592–600.

30. Chwastiak LA, Rosenheck RA, McEnvoy JP *et al*. Interrelationships of psychiatric symptom severity, medical comorbidity, and functioning in schizophrenia. *Psychiatric Services* 2006; 57:1102–1109.

31. Elmer PJ, Obarzanek E, Vollmer WM *et al*. Effects of comprehensive lifestyle modification on diet, weight, physical fitness, and blood pressure control: 18-month results of a randomized trial. *Ann Intern Med* 2006; 144:485–495.

32. Daniels SR, Long B, Crow S *et al*. Cardiovascular effects of sibutramine in the treatment of obese adolescents: results of a randomized, double-blind, placebo-controlled study. *Pediatrics* 2007; 120:e147–e157.

33. Flynn JT, Daniels SR. Pharmacologic treatment of hypertension in children and adolescents. *J Pediatr* 2006; 149:746–754.

34. Woroniecki RP, Flynn JT. How are hypertensive children evaluated and managed? A survey of North American pediatric nephrologists. *Pediatr Nephrol* 2005; 20:791–797.

35. Sieber US, von Vigier RO, Sforzini C *et al*. How good is blood pressure control among treated hypertensive children and adolescents? *J Hypertens* 2003; 21:633–637.

36. McMahan CA, Gidding SS, Malcom GT *et al*. Pathobiological determinants of atherosclerosis in youth risk scores are associated with early and advanced atherosclerosis. *Pediatrics* 2006; 118:1447–1455.

10

Is there a role for α-blockers in the treatment of hypertension?

J. L. Pool, A. A. Taylor

BACKGROUND

THE ROLE OF α-ADRENOCEPTORS IN CONTROL OF VASCULAR SMOOTH MUSCLE TONE

Alpha-adrenoceptors in conjunction with β-adrenoceptors and dopaminergic receptors are the adrenergic receptors that modulate sympathetic nervous system (SNS) control of vascular function. Alpha-adrenoceptors participate in the physiological regulation of vascular resistance and also play a role in hypertension [1–3] and other cardiovascular (CV) disorders, including myocardial hypertrophy [4], obstructive sleep apnea [5] and metabolic syndrome [6]. Activation of these G-protein coupled receptors, ubiquitously distributed in vascular smooth muscle of blood vessels, the prostate gland, and on sympathetic nerve terminals, promotes vasoconstriction and prostate smooth muscle contraction while reducing sympathetic neuronal release of norepinephrine. To understand the role of α adrenoceptors and the modulation of receptor function in hypertension by pharmacological antagonists of these receptors, it is necessary to be familiar with the contributions of the SNS to the development of hypertension [3, 7–9].

Arterial pressure is regulated by changes in cardiac output and/or systemic vascular resistance. Modulation of vascular smooth muscle tone in arteries plays a prominent role in the control of vascular resistance whereas smooth muscle tone in veins participates in the regulation of venous capacitance. In addition to the blood vessels, the urinary bladder, penis and prostate also have smooth muscle cells innervated by sympathetic and parasympathetic neurons that participate in the regulation of micturition, erection and ejaculation [10, 11]. As noted later, the SNS influences on lower urinary tract function play an important role in benign prostatic hyperplasia (BPH) [12] and lower urinary tract symptoms (LUTS) [13], both common conditions among older males with hypertension.

THE SYMPATHETIC NERVOUS SYSTEM IN HYPERTENSION

Increased SNS activity has been documented in persons with high blood pressure (BP). This increased SNS activity promotes vasoconstriction and thereby increases total peripheral vascular resistance. Studies in both borderline and mild hypertension have observed an

James L. Pool, MD, Professor of Medicine and Pharmacology, Baylor College of Medicine, Houston, Texas, USA.

Addison A. Taylor, MD, PhD, Professor of Medicine and Pharmacology, Division of Hypertension and Clinical Pharmacology, Section on Cardiovascular Research, Department of Medicine, Baylor College of Medicine, Houston, Texas, USA.

Table 10.1 Alpha-1 adrenoceptor subtypes (adapted with permission from [17]).

Native receptors	Cloned receptors	Cloned receptors (historical)	Human chromosome location
	1995 Classification		
α_{1A}	α_{1a}	α_{1a}	C8
α_{1B}	α_{1b}	α_{1b}	C5
α_{1D}	α_{1d}	$\alpha_{1a/d}$, α_{1a}	C20

increased cardiac β-adrenergic drive with a high cardiac output and faster heart rate, as well as an increased vascular α-adrenergic drive. A longitudinal study over 20 years showed the gradual transformation of such borderline hypertensive patients to established hypertension with normal cardiac output and increased vascular resistance [14]. Mechanisms that underlie this transition from a high cardiac output state to one of high vascular resistance involve modifications of SNS receptors and a significant role for α-adrenoceptors. There is functional down-regulation of β-adrenergic responsiveness in the heart [15] plus alterations in vascular anatomy and function [3] followed by a steady increase in vascular resistance. An exaggerated response of blood vessels to adrenergic and non-adrenergic vasoconstrictors develops that likely contributes to the progressive increase in vascular resistance during this evolutionary phase of hypertension [16].

THE SUBTYPES OF α-ADRENOCEPTORS

Most vasomotor neurons are noradrenergic with the neurotransmitter norepinephrine producing vasoconstriction by acting on a specific type of vascular smooth muscle transmembrane receptor, the α-adrenoceptor. Six α-adrenoceptor subtypes, which have been designated α_{1A}, α_{1B}, α_{1D}, α_{2A}, α_{2B}, and α_{2C} , are now identified [17]. Their chromosomal location is noted in Table 10.1. The vascular endothelium expresses at least two different α-adrenoceptor subtypes (α_{2A}, α_{2C}) which, along with β- and DA-adrenoceptor subtypes, actively participate in the regulation of vascular tone. The specific roles for each of these multiple subtypes of adrenoceptors in the regulation of BP are not completely defined.

SELECTIVE POST-SYNAPTIC α_1-ADRENOCEPTOR BLOCKADE

When stimulated, α_1-adrenoceptors, located post-synaptically on smooth muscle, produce arterial vasoconstriction. Sympathetic over-activity in hypertension results in an excess stimulation of postsynaptic α_1-adrenoceptors. Consequently, there emerged a sound therapeutic rationale for the use of selective α_1-blockers in the treatment of hypertension. By selectively inhibiting the vascular α_1-adrenoceptor and thereby inhibiting the receptor-mediated response to norepinephrine, these agents reduce BP via a decrease in peripheral vascular resistance [18]. The ensuing reduction in BP pressure is accomplished with little to no change in central hemodynamic parameters, such as heart rate, stroke index or cardiac index.

AN OVERVIEW OF α-ADRENOCEPTOR ANTAGONISTS

The non-selective α-adrenoceptor antagonists, phentolamine and phenoxybenzamine, which bind to both α_1 and α_2 receptors, were the first compounds in this class to be used for BP reduction. Phenoxybenzamine is a non-competitive, non-selective α-blocker that is now

Table 10.2 Pharmacokinetics of selective α_1-adrenergic antagonists.

Drug	Daily dose (mg)	Frequency of dosing	Bioavailability	Half-life	Urinary excretion
Prazosin	2–20	2–3/day	44–69	2.5–4	10
Terazosin	1–20	1/day	90	12	10
Doxazosin	1–16	1/day	65	19–22	5

reserved for the pre-operative management of pheo-chromocytoma-related hypertension. Non-selective α-blockade means that presynaptic α_2-receptors, which reduce the release of norepinephrine, are inhibited and the important negative feedback mechanism is also blocked. Phentolamine is a competitive, short-acting, parenterally administered non-selective α-blocker used almost exclusively for urgent severe forms of hypertension prompted by excessive catecholamine release [19].

Alternatively, selective α_1-blockers lower BP primarily by post-synaptic α_1-adrenoceptor blockade. In this respect, selective α_1-blockers differ from the non-selective α-blockers, phentolamine and phenoxybenzamine [20]. Importantly, the stimulation of pre-synaptic α_2-adrenoceptors inhibits norepinephrine release. Non-selective α-blockade prevents this inhibition and causes α_2-receptors to increase norepinephrine release with β-adrenoceptor mediated tachycardia, enhanced renin secretion, and attenuation of post-synaptic α_1-inhibition. In fact, selective blockade of these pre-synaptic α_2-adrenoceptors with a drug such as yohimbine can increase BP. As a result of these pharmacodynamic consequences of non-selective α-adrenoceptor blockade, attempts to treat essential hypertension and symptomatic BPH with drugs of this type were unsuccessful.

In contrast to the non-selective drugs, the selective α_1-blockers, which include the three antihypertensive agents marketed in the USA, doxazosin, prazosin and terazosin, reduce vascular tone in capacitance vessels as well as resistance vessels to provide a balance of preload and afterload reduction thus avoiding vasodilation (afterload reduction) without venodilation (preload reduction), which would in kind promote an increase in cardiac output and heart rate.

Prazosin was the first selective α-blocker and is a compound with a high affinity for the α_1-adrenoreceptor. When given as an immediate-release formulation it has a rapid onset of action, a feature that probably accounts for the higher rate of syncope and orthostatic hypotension compared with doxazosin and terazosin. The individual members of the α_1-adrenergic antagonist class are pharmacologically distinct. Prazosin has a relatively short duration of action and should be given at least twice daily (Table 10.2) [21]. Terazosin and doxazosin have longer half-lives and can be administered once daily. Doxazosin can be administered at bedtime with its pattern of slow absorption allowing for a maximal effect on the early morning surge in BP [22]. In general, α_1-adrenergic antagonists should be used cautiously in children or in pregnancy since the efficacy and/or safety of these compounds have not been evaluated in these patient types [21].

TREATMENT OF HYPERTENSION WITH α_1-ADRENOCEPTOR ANTAGONISTS

Clinical studies have shown that α_1-blockers lower BP through a reduction in vascular resistance without significant effects on heart rate, cardiac output or central hemodynamic parameters in hypertensive patients [23]. In normotensive subjects who have normal sympathetic tone and peripheral vascular resistance, the BP effects of these compounds are not clinically significant, which has contributed to their utility in the treatment of conditions other than hypertension, such as BPH and Raynaud's Disease. Prazosin, terazosin and doxazosin are all effective antihypertensive agents, whether used as monotherapy or as part of a regimen of multiple antihypertensive drugs. Because of their longer duration of action, doxazosin and terazosin have generally replaced prazosin in the treatment of both hypertension and BPH.

Alpha$_1$-adrenergic antagonists are most effective in low and medium plasma renin activity states. When used to treat hypertension, the effects of these compounds are additive to those of ACE inhibitors, angiotensin receptor antagonists, β-blockers, calcium channel blockers, diuretics, and direct-acting vasodilators. About 50% of patients with stage I essential hypertension treated with monotherapy in placebo-controlled trials will achieve diastolic BPs <90 mmHg but fewer will achieve systolic BP values of <140 mmHg [24]. In large placebo-controlled studies of hypertensive patients, doxazosin or terazosin once daily lowered BP at trough (24 h after dosing) by ~10/8 mmHg compared to placebo in the standing position and ~9/5 mmHg in the supine position. Age, race and gender do not influence the BP response to selective α$_1$-blockers. For over a decade of clinical practice α$_1$-blockers have had their widest application as a component of multiple drug regimens for the treatment of moderate to severe hypertension [25]. Although less pronounced than what is observed with potent direct vasodilators, selective α$_1$-blockers promote sodium and water retention. Use of a diuretic prevents such fluid retention and therein can markedly enhance the antihypertensive effect of these drugs.

IMPACT OF ALLHAT ON THE TREATMENT OF HYPERTENSION WITH α-BLOCKERS

The Antihypertensive Lipid Lowering Heart Attack Trial (ALLHAT) was the first clinical trial to examine the effects of selective α$_1$-blockers on morbidity and mortality. This federally sponsored clinical trial enrolled over 42 000 hypertensive patients over age 55 years who also had at least one other risk factor for coronary artery disease (CAD), and assigned them to treatment with one of the following drugs: the thiazide-type diuretic – chlorthalidone, the angiotensin converting enzyme (ACE) inhibitor – lisinopril, the dihydropyridine calcium channel antagonist amlodipine, or the selective α$_1$-blocker doxazosin. The question addressed by this CV events trial was whether each of these "newer" drugs was superior to chlorthalidone for reducing fatal and non-fatal myocardial infarction (MI). Of note, ALLHAT did not include a placebo group and there was no washout period for patients taking antihypertensive drugs at time of enrollment into the trial.

Although the trial was not expected to conclude until 2002, an independent data and safety monitoring board recommended that the doxazosin arm of the trial be discontinued after an interim analysis in January 2000 revealed comparable risk of coronary heart disease (CHD) death and non-fatal MI but an increased risk of combined cardiovascular disease (CVD) events, particularly congestive heart failure (CHF), in the cohort of patients treated with a doxazosin-based regimen compared to a chlorthalidone-based regimen [26, 27]. As observed in Figure 10.1, patients taking doxazosin had a significantly higher relative risk of stroke, combined CVD, angina, coronary revascularization and CHF. Congestive heart failure risk in the doxazosin arm was nearly twice (8.13% vs. 4.45%) that of the chlorthalidone arm. The investigators speculated that the 3/0 mmHg higher average systolic/diastolic BP (doxazosin vs. chlorthalidone) could account for only 10–20% of the observed difference in CHF rates based on extrapolation of data from the Systolic Hypertension in the Elderly Program (SHEP) [28] and Systolic Hypertension in Europe (Syst-Eur) [29] placebo-controlled clinical trials that included older patients with isolated systolic hypertension. In contrast, the authors noted that this same difference in BP was sufficient to account for most of the difference in stroke and angina rates in the two groups.

As noted previously, the above findings are subject to a variety of interpretations that have implications for the inclusion of selective α$_1$-blockers as part of a multi-drug regimen

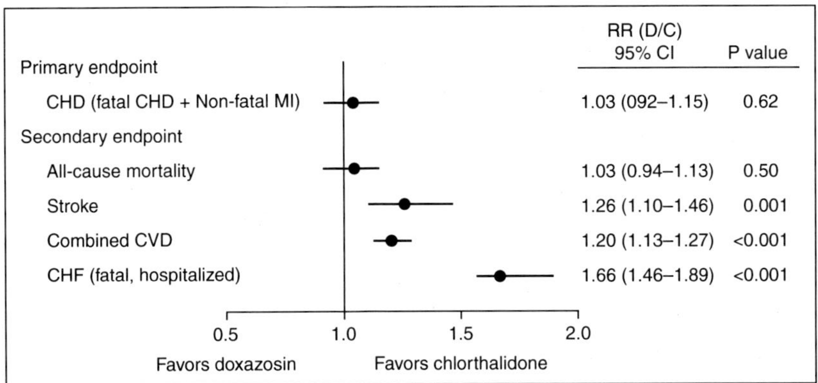

Figure 10.1 The principle outcomes of ALLHAT for the α-blocker (doxazosin) treatment arm vs. diuretic (chlorthalidone) treatment arm are shown for the primary CHD endpoint and the four major secondary endpoints (with permission from [22]). CI = confidence interval; D/C = doxazosin compared to chlorthalidone; MI = myocardial infarction; RR = risk ratio.

to control BP. One interesting consideration is that the observed risk of CHF in the chlorthalidone versus placebo treated population (2.3 vs. 4.4%; ratio 0.52) in SHEP was similar to that of the chlorthalidone vs. doxazosin-treated cohorts (4.45 vs. 8.13%; ratio 0.55) in ALLHAT and better than the nitrendipine vs. placebo-treated arms of Syst-Eur (8.7 vs. 6.2; ratio 0.71). One could interpret these data as suggesting that doxazosin is less likely to be causing CHF as chlorthalidone is to blunt or prevent its symptoms. Furthermore, patients taking 1–2 medications but with still inadequately controlled BP at the time of enrollment into ALLHAT could have drugs like diuretics discontinued and doxazosin started with no transition period of observation. Diuretics are of course an integral component of any CHF therapeutic regimen and loss of chlorthalidone in a patient with incipient CHF could have deleterious clinical consequences. The early divergence in the cumulative event rate curves for chlorthalidone and doxazosin would be consistent with such a scenario, especially when the additional drugs that could be added to the doxazosin regimen if the BP was not controlled were atenolol, reserpine or clonidine, followed by hydralazine. Compared to baseline values, doxazosin did lower BP 14/10 mmHg and chlorthalidone 16/10 mmHg during the fourth year of treatment (Figure 10.2).

The results of meta-analyses [30, 31] of clinical trial outcomes emphasize the importance of BP reduction in reducing fatal and non-fatal hypertension-related CV events. Doxazosin is clearly capable of lowering BP in hypertensive patients. As part of a multi-drug regimen that might include a diuretic, ACE inhibitor or ARB, calcium channel blocker or beta blocker, for the patient whose BP is difficult to control, additional BP reduction is achieved with addition of doxazosin [32].

IMPACT OF ALLHAT TRIAL RESULTS ON α_1-BLOCKER USE

Subsequent to the publication of the ALLHAT comparison of doxazosin and chlorthalidone demonstrating that the diuretic was superior to the α_1 blocker in reducing combined CV events (particularly CHF, in older hypertensives with increased CV risk) the hypertension management guidelines of several countries were modified to recommend that α_1-blockers not be used as first line treatment. These recommendations applied to all hypertensive patients, even though the ALLHAT study was not designed to investigate the use of α_1-blockers for:

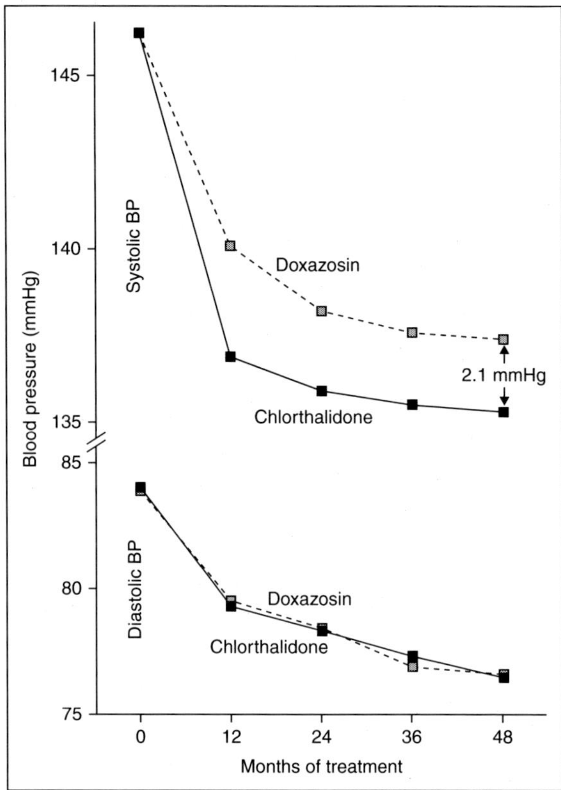

Figure 10.2 Mean systolic and diastolic blood pressures (BPs) in ALLHAT are shown at baseline and four annual visits. Diastolic BP is controlled equally, but there is consistently a 2–3 mmHg higher systolic BP in the doxazosin group at all treatment visits (with permission from [22]).

1. Younger hypertensive subjects or hypertensives with a lesser CHD risk factor profile.
2. Diuretic-based combination therapy for the treatment of hypertension.
3. Combined treatment of hypertension and BPH.
4. Treatment of normotensive patients with BPH, where α_1-blockers remain the best monotherapy for the control of symptoms.

In spring 2000 as a result of early, unfavorable results from ALLHAT, α-blockers were no longer recommended as first line treatment for hypertension in high-risk patients. Stafford *et al* [33] tracked trends in α-blocker prescriptions filled by community pharmacies and reports of α-blocker use in patient encounters with office-based physicians from 1996 to 2002. The authors used United States data from two sources:

1. α-blocker prescription orders reported in the National Prescription Audit, a random, computerized sample of about 20 000 of 29 000 pharmacies.
2. Office-based physician α-blocker prescribing patterns reported in the National Disease and Therapeutic Index, a random sample of about 3500 physician offices.

The researchers found that there had been steady increases in new α-blocker prescriptions, dispensed prescriptions, and physician prescribing from 1996 through 1999. But, there was a moderate reversal in these trends following the early termination of the doxazosin-based therapy arm in ALLHAT. Between 1999 and 2002, new annual α-blocker prescription orders declined by 26% from 5.15 million to 3.79 million, dispensed prescriptions by 22% from 17.2 million to 13.4 million, and physician-reported drug use by 54% from 2.26 million to 1.03 million.

INEFFECTIVE FOR TREATMENT OF HEART FAILURE

Alpha blockers have not shown sustained benefits in chronic CHF. Mortality from left ventricular dysfunction is not improved by selective α_1-blockers. In the 1986 Veterans Administration Cooperative Study [34], which examined the effect of vasodilator therapy in chronic CHF, mortality in the prazosin treatment group was similar to that in the placebo group. Furthermore, chronic therapy in CHF with the α_1-blocker (doxazosin) plus the β-blocker (metoprolol) produced identical effects as those seen in patients receiving β-blocker therapy alone [35].

METABOLIC EFFECTS

Selective α_1-blockers have proven beneficial effects on the lipid profiles of hypertensive patients. Several clinical trials have demonstrated reductions of total cholesterol, low density lipoprotein (LDL) cholesterol, and triglycerides, and increased levels of high density lipoprotein (HDL) cholesterol and the ratio of HDL cholesterol to total cholesterol [36]. A recent meta-analysis of 22 controlled clinical trials reported similar effects of selective α_1-blockers in hypertensive patients with type 2 diabetes mellitus [37]. In addition, doxazosin was noted to improve insulin sensitivity and lower fasting glucose and serum insulin levels. In hypertensive patients with baseline values similar to the general population, doxazosin produced small reductions in total serum cholesterol (2–3%), LDL cholesterol (4%), and a similarly small increase in the HDL to total cholesterol ratio (4%). These modifications of the serum lipid profile are the result of several different mechanisms [38]. These mechanisms include an increase in LDL cholesterol receptor number, a decrease in LDL cholesterol synthesis, stimulation of lipoprotein lipase activity, reduction of very low density lipoprotein (VLDL) cholesterol synthesis and secretion, and a reduction in the absorption of dietary cholesterol [39].

The favorable metabolic profile of the selective α_1-blockers might be expected to translate into improved CV outcomes in hypertensive patients with concomitant dyslipidemia or at least into improvement in surrogate markers of these CV outcomes compared to antihypertensive drugs like diuretics and β-blockers that have less favorable metabolic profiles. Only a limited number of studies have examined either outcomes or surrogate markers. In a recent open-label study of hypertensive patients with impaired glucose tolerance whose BPs were uncontrolled on other therapies, doxazosin add-on therapy was associated with improved BP control and with a reduction in the 10-year Framingham CHD risk score of 17% after 16 weeks of therapy [32]. The duration of the study was too short, however, to ascertain if the changes in lipids and in glucose metabolism might have beneficially impacted CV outcomes in this small cohort. Measurements of intimal-medial thickness (IMT) of the carotid artery by B-mode ultrasonography have been proposed as a surrogate marker for the progression or regression of atherosclerosis [40]. In a clinical trial comparing doxazosin and hydrochlorothiazide (HCTZ) on arterial wall thickness in men with hypertension and hypercholesterolemia, both drugs reduced IMT in the femoral and carotid arteries an equivalent amount after 3 years of therapy, despite an improvement in the lipid profile of patients treated with doxazosin but not HCTZ [41].

There was no difference in the risk of CHD death and non-fatal MI between the doxazosin and chlorthalidone arms of the ALLHAT trial despite poorer BP control in the doxazosin group, but the impact of changes in lipid profiles or indices of glucose metabolism in these two treatment groups is not yet appreciated since these data are to date not published [26]. Thus, these is currently no compelling evidence that improved indices of glucose tolerance and better lipid profiles with selective α_1-blocker therapy in hypertensive patients, with or without diabetes, leads to a greater reduction in either surrogate markers of atherosclerosis or CV events than antihypertensive drugs that are absent those metabolic characteristics. Conversely, there are no data to suggest that the selective α_1-blockers are more likely to accelerate the progression of atherosclerosis than other antihypertensive agents. Thus, they should be considered as part of a multi-drug regimen to achieve goal BPs when other drug combinations have proven inadequate.

ALPHA-BLOCKERS FOR THE MANAGEMENT OF BPH

Any discussion of the use of selective α_1-blockers for the treatment of hypertension would not be complete without some mention of their frequent use in men with lower urinary tract obstructive symptoms (LUTS). For men over the age of 60 years, LUTS associated with BPH and obstruction occurs in up to 70% [42]. This is the age group of men in whom the prevalence of hypertension is also approximately 70% [43]. Prior to the availability of effective medical management, men with bothersome LUTS were observed for variable lengths of time until they were considered suitable candidates for transurethral prostatectomy (TURP). In the early 1970s, selective α_1-blockers emerged as an effective treatment option for LUTS secondary to BPH [44]. Such therapy with selective α_1-blockers soon emerged as the major clinical option in the management of BPH including men with mild to severe LUTS. There was a subsequent increase in prescriptions for selective α_1-blocker medical therapy and a decline in TURP as a therapy choice [45]. Much of the early use of selective α_1-blocker therapy for the medical therapy of BPH was off-label. In that regard, terazosin was approved for treatment of hypertension in 1987 and, in 1994, it was approved for treatment of LUTS, followed by approval of doxazosin for both indications. Finasteride, the 5-α reductase inhibitor, which blocks the conversion of testosterone to dihydrotestosterone, was approved in 1992 for the treatment of BPH. However, α-blockers retained their popularity because they have proven to be more effective in the short-term relief of LUTS than is finasteride. From 59% to 86% of men using selective α_1-blockers will typically experience a decrease in symptoms within 2 to 3 weeks of initiating therapy [42]. Terazosin and doxazosin typically improve urinary flow rate by 2–2.5 ml/min.

Clinically, tamsulosin introduced the concept of uroselectivity with α_1-blockade. Targeting the α_{1a} and α_{1b}-adrenoceptors in the bladder neck and prostate, tamsulosin achieves greater effect on the prostate and a similar degree of improvement in both urine flow rates and symptoms with little to no BP effect compared to non-selective agents [46]. Tamsulosin is typically not dose-titrated in that the incidence of retrograde ejaculation with higher doses of tamsulosin (>0.4 mg/day) approaches 20%. In addition, it and other α-blockers have been implicated in the intra-operative floppy iris syndrome noted during cataract surgery, which includes fluttering and billowing of the iris stroma, propensity for iris prolapse, and constriction of the pupil [47]. This syndrome typically occurs when tamsulosin therapy is concurrent with surgery but has developed during surgery even months after discontinuation of tamsulosin.

The Veterans Affairs (VA) Cooperative BPH Study [48] in 1996 was the first large-scale study (n = 1229) to compare an α-blocker (terazosin), a 5-α reductase inhibitor (finasteride), and the combination of these two agents for the improvement of LUTS and urine flow rate in BPH. In this 1-year VA trial, terazosin achieved greater improvement in symptoms and flow rate than did finasteride, whose effect was similar to that of placebo. Furthermore, the combination of terazosin and finasteride was not better than an α-blocker alone. However, the 4-year Proscar® (finasteride) Long-Term Efficacy and Safety Study (PLESS) [49] with

3040 men reported the impact of finasteride alone compared to placebo on disease progression defined as acute urinary retention (AUR) and BPH surgery. Finasteride reduced the incidence of AUR by 57% and surgery for BPH by 55% compared with placebo, which established a different role for finasteride in the long-term management of BPH than is the case for selective α-blockers. Men with moderate to severe symptoms and an enlarged prostate respond best to finasteride therapy. Men with little or no enlargement of the prostate gland are less likely to experience symptomatic improvement with finasteride. Alternatively, the size of the prostate does not predict improvement in LUTS symptoms during selective α-blocker therapy.

In 2003, the Medical Therapy of Prostatic Symptoms (MTOPS) Trial [42] with 3047 men over 4.5 years established a role for combination drug therapy with an α-blocker and finasteride. The "overall risk of clinical progression" – defined as an increase from baseline of ≥4 points in the American Urologic Association (AUA) symptom score, acute urinary retention, urinary incontinence, renal insufficiency, or recurrent urinary tract infections – was significantly reduced by doxazosin 39%, finasteride 34%, and the combination of doxazosin + finasteride 66%, as compared to placebo. Long-term combination therapy with doxazosin and finasteride was safe and reduced the risk of overall clinical progression of BPH more than did treatment with either drug alone. Combination therapy and finasteride alone reduced the long-term risk of AUR and the need for invasive BPH therapy. The principal effect of doxazosin on progression was prevention of a 4-point rise in the AUA symptom score.

These recent long-term, large clinical trials of medical therapy for BPH have clarified treatment options. Alpha-blockers offer the best monotherapy for symptom relief of LUTS. Among the available selective α-blockers, their effects on symptoms and flow rate are similar. Finasteride prevents disease progression, whether defined by symptoms, AUR, or surgery. Finally, combination therapy with an α-blocker + finasteride is the most effective treatment for BPH symptoms and disease progression and the ideal candidates for combination therapy have moderate to severe symptoms and prostatic enlargement.

ADVERSE DRUG EFFECTS

Selective α_1-antagonists are generally well-tolerated with a few common effects. In placebo-controlled trials, the symptoms that most commonly caused discontinuation of selective α_1-antagonist therapy were asthenia (2%), nasal congestion (2%), and dizziness (1%) [24, 50, 51]. Generally, there is a limited drug–dose relationship for these particular adverse effects. Dizziness secondary to α_1-blockers is not entirely understood, since patients can experience this sensation without documented postural hypotension. However, a major precaution is the so-called "first dose phenomenon", which is severe, symptomatic orthostatic hypotension, which usually occurs within the first 90 minutes after the first dose or when the dose is increased rapidly. If the patient has prior treatment with one or more agents (especially a diuretic, β-blocker, or verapamil), additional caution with the first dose is advisable. Syncope is uncommon, occurring in <1% of patients when an initial, small dose (1 mg or less) was taken at bedtime as monotherapy.

Selective α_1-blockers cause salt and water retention, which can significantly attenuate their BP lowering effect [52]. Such sodium retention is dose-dependent and occurs perhaps because plasma renin activity and plasma aldosterone do not suppress as completely with α_1-adrenergic antagonists as they do with other adrenergic-inhibiting drugs. Males should be cautioned that the combination of an α_1-blocker and sildenafil (Viagra®), tadalafil (Cialis®) or vardenafil (Levitra®) can occasionally cause marked hypertension [53]. Erectile dysfunction is not a common finding in α_1-blocker-treated males. Post-menopausal women with pelvic relaxation syndrome and individuals with certain types of urinary bladder dysfunction can develop urinary incontinence as the result of α_1-blocker-mediated relaxation of the bladder outlet [54].

There are no clinically important adverse effects on common laboratory tests or renal function with α_1-blocker therapy. In placebo-controlled trials, a greater percentage of α_1-blocker patients have small decreases in hematocrit, hemoglobin, white blood cell count, total serum protein and albumin levels from baseline values. Except for the white blood cell count, these changes have been attributed to hemodilution secondary to mild fluid retention. The reduction of white blood cell counts remains unexplained with α_1-blockers but individual reductions have been small and prolonged drug treatment has not been associated with progressive white blood cell count reductions.

REFERENCES

1.   Victor RG, Shafiq MM. Sympathetic neural mechanisms in human hypertension. *Curr Hypertens Rep* 2008; 10:241–247.
2.   Mark AL. The sympathetic nervous system in hypertension: a potential long-term regulator of arterial pressure. *J Hypertens (Suppl)* 1996; 14:S159–S165.
3.   Somers VK, Anderson EA, Mark AL. Sympathetic neural mechanisms in human hypertension. *Curr Opin Nephrol Hypertens* 1993; 2:96–105.
4.   Tarone G, Lembo G. Molecular interplay between mechanical and humoral signaling in cardiac hypertrophy. *Trends Mol Med* 2003; 9:376–382.
5.   Okcay A, Somers VK, Caples SM. Obstructive sleep apnea and hypertension. *J Clin Hypertens (Greenwich)* 2008; 10:549–555.
6.   Straznicky NE, Eikelis N, Lambert EA, Esler MD. Mediators of sympathetic activation in metabolic syndrome obesity. *Curr Hypertens Rep* 2008; 10:440–447.
7.   Sivertsson R. Structural adaptation in borderline hypertension. *Hypertension* 1984; 6:III103–III107.
8.   Anderson EA, Sinkey CA, Lawton WJ, Mark AL. Elevated sympathetic nerve activity in borderline hypertensive humans. Evidence from direct intraneural recordings. *Hypertension* 1989; 14:177–183.
9.   Julius S, Majahalme S. The changing face of sympathetic overactivity in hypertension. *Ann Med* 2000; 32:365–370.
10. Andersson KE. Bladder activation: afferent mechanisms. *Urology* 2002; 59(5 suppl 1):43–50.
11. Andersson KE. Treatment of the overactive bladder: possible central nervous system drug targets. *Urology* 2002; 59(5 suppl 1):18–24.
12. Berry SJ, Coffey DS, Walsh PC, Ewing LL. The development of human benign prostatic hyperplasia with age. *J Urol* 1984; 132:474–479.
13. Chute CG, Panser LA, Girman CJ *et al*. The prevalence of prostatism: a population-based survey of urinary symptoms. *J Urol* 1993; 150:85–89.
14. Lund-Johansen P. Central haemodynamics in essential hypertension at rest and during exercise: a 20-year follow-up study. *J Hypertens (Suppl)* 1989; 7:S52–S55.
15. Trimarco B, Volpe M, Ricciardelli B *et al*. Studies of the mechanisms underlying impairment of beta-adrenoceptor-mediated effects in human hypertension. *Hypertension* 1983; 5:584–590.
16. Cain AE, Khalil RA. Pathophysiology of essential hypertension: role of the pump, the vessel, and the kidney. *Semin Nephrol* 2002; 22:3–16.
17. Hieble JP. Subclassification and nomenclature of alpha- and beta-adrenoceptors. *Curr Top Med Chem* 2007; 7:129–134.
18. Lund-Johansen P, Omvik P. Acute and chronic hemodynamic effects of drugs with different actions on adrenergic receptors: a comparison between alpha blockers and different types of beta blockers with and without vasodilating effect. *Cardiovasc Drugs Ther* 1991; 5:605–615.
19. Kincaid-Smith P. Vasodilator drugs in the treatment of hypertension. *Med J Aust* 1985; 142:450–453.
20. Davey M. Mechanism of alpha blockade for blood pressure control. *Am J Cardiol* 1987; 59:18G–28G.
21. Sica DA. Alpha-adrenergic blockers: current usage considerations. *J Clin Hyper Greenwich* 2005; 7:757–762.
22. Kawano Y, Tochikubo O, Watanabe Y *et al*. Doxazosin suppresses the morning increase in blood pressure and sympathetic nervous activity in patients with essential hypertension. *Hypertens Res* 1997; 20:149–156.
23. Lund-Johansen P, Hjermann I, Iversen BM, Thaulow E. Selective alpha-1 inhibitors: first- or second-line antihypertensive agents? *Cardiology* 1993; 83:150–159.
24. Pool JL. Terazosin. In: Messerli FH (ed.). *Cardiovascular Drug Therapy*, 2nd edition. W.B. Saunders Co., Philadelphia, 1996, pp 665–673.

25. Campo C, Segura J, Roldan C *et al*. Doxazosin GITS versus hydrochlorothiazide as add-on therapy in patients with uncontrolled hypertension. *Blood Press (suppl)* 2003; 2:16–21.
26. Major cardiovascular events in hypertensive patients randomized to doxazosin vs chlorthalidone: the Antihypertensive and Lipid-Lowering Treatment to Prevent Heart Attack Trial (ALLHAT). ALLHAT Collaborative Research Group. *JAMA* 2000; 283:1967–1975.
27. Davis BR, Cutler JA, Furberg CD *et al*. Relationship of antihypertensive treatment regimens and change in blood pressure to risk for heart failure in hypertensive patients randomly assigned to doxazosin or chlorthalidone: further analyses from the Antihypertensive and Lipid-Lowering Treatment to Prevent Heart Attack Trial. *Ann Intern Med* 2002; 137(5 Part 1):313–320.
28. Prevention of stroke by antihypertensive drug treatment in older persons with isolated systolic hypertension. Final results of the Systolic Hypertension in the Elderly Program (SHEP). SHEP Cooperative Research Group. *JAMA* 1991; 265:3255–3264.
29. Staessen JA, Fagard R, Thijs L *et al*. Randomised double-blind comparison of placebo and active treatment for older patients with isolated systolic hypertension. The Systolic Hypertension in Europe (Syst-Eur) Trial Investigators. *Lancet* 1997; 350:757–764.
30. Staessen JA, Wang JG, Thijs L. Cardiovascular protection and blood pressure reduction: a meta-analysis. *Lancet* 2001; 358:1305–1315.
31. Verdecchia P, Reboldi G, Angeli F *et al*. Angiotensin-converting enzyme inhibitors and calcium channel blockers for coronary heart disease and stroke prevention. *Hypertension* 2005; 46:386–392.
32. Pessina AC, Ciccariello L, Perrone F *et al*. Clinical efficacy and tolerability of alpha-blocker doxazosin as add-on therapy in patients with hypertension and impaired glucose metabolism. *Nutr Metab Cardiovasc Dis* 2006; 16:137–147.
33. Stafford RS, Furberg CD, Finkelstein SN, Cockburn IM, Alehegn T, Ma J. Impact of clinical trial results on national trends in alpha-blocker prescribing, 1996–2002. *JAMA* 2004; 291:54–62.
34. Cohn JN, Archibald DG, Ziesche S *et al*. Effect of vasodilator therapy on mortality in chronic congestive heart failure. Results of a Veterans Administration Cooperative Study. *N Engl J Med* 1986; 314:1547–1552.
35. Kukin ML, Kalman J, Mannino M, Freudenberger R, Buchholz C, Ocampo O. Combined alpha–beta blockade (doxazosin plus metoprolol) compared with beta blockade alone in chronic congestive heart failure. *Am J Cardiol* 1996; 77:486–491.
36. Cubeddu LX, Pool JL, Bloomfield R *et al*. Effect of doxazosin monotherapy on blood pressure and plasma lipids in patients with essential hypertension. *Am J Hypertens* 1988; 1:158–167.
37. Glanz M, Garber AJ, Mancia G, Levenstein M. Meta-analysis of studies using selective alpha1-blockers in patients with hypertension and type 2 diabetes. *Int J Clin Pract* 2001; 55:694–701.
38. Pool JL, Lenz ML, Taylor AA. Alpha 1-adrenoreceptor blockade and the molecular basis of lipid metabolism alterations. *J Hum Hypertens* 1990; 4(suppl 3):23–33.
39. Pool JL. Effects of doxazosin on serum lipids: a review of the clinical data and molecular basis for altered lipid metabolism. *Am Heart J* 1991; 121:251–259.
40. Hulthe J, Wikstrand J, Emanuelsson H, Wiklund O, de Feyter PJ, Wendelhag I. Atherosclerotic changes in the carotid artery bulb as measured by B-mode ultrasound are associated with the extent of coronary atherosclerosis. *Stroke* 1997; 28:1189–1194.
41. Hoogerbrugge N, de Groot E, de Heide LH *et al*. Doxazosin and hydrochlorothiazide equally affect arterial wall thickness in hypertensive males with hypercholesterolaemia (the DAPHNE study). Doxazosin Atherosclerosis Progression Study in Hypertensives in The Netherlands. *Neth J Med* 2002; 60:354–361.
42. McConnell JD, Roehrborn CG, Bautista OM *et al*. The long-term effect of doxazosin, finasteride, and combination therapy on the clinical progression of benign prostatic hyperplasia. *N Engl J Med* 2003; 349:2387–2398.
43. Rosamond W, Flegal K, Furie K *et al*. Heart disease and stroke statistics – 2008 update: a report from the American Heart Association Statistics Committee and Stroke Statistics Subcommittee. *Circulation* 2008; 117:e25–e146.
44. Kirby RS, Pool JL. Alpha adrenoceptor blockade in the treatment of benign prostatic hyperplasia: past, present and future. *Br J Urol* 1997; 80:521–532.
45. Edwards JL. Diagnosis and management of benign prostatic hyperplasia. *Am Fam Physician* 2008; 77:1403–1410.
46. Nargund VH, Grey AD. Tamsulosin MR and OCAS (modified release and oral controlled absorption system): current therapeutic uses. *Expert Opin Pharmacother* 2008; 9:813–824.

47. Cantrell MA, Bream-Rouwenhorst HR, Steffensmeier A, Hemerson P, Rogers M, Stamper B. Intraoperative floppy iris syndrome associated with alpha1-adrenergic receptor antagonists. *Ann Pharmacother* 2008; 42:558–563.

48. Lepor H, Williford WO, Barry MJ *et al*. The efficacy of terazosin, finasteride, or both in benign prostatic hyperplasia. Veterans Affairs Cooperative Studies Benign Prostatic Hyperplasia Study Group. *N Engl J Med* 1996; 335:533–539.

49. McConnell JD, Bruskewitz R, Walsh P *et al*. The effect of finasteride on the risk of acute urinary retention and the need for surgical treatment among men with benign prostatic hyperplasia. Finasteride Long-Term Efficacy and Safety Study Group. *N Engl J Med* 1998; 338:557–563.

50. Neutel JM, Taylor SH, Smith DGH, Pool JL. Doxazosin. In: Messerli FH (ed.). *Cardiovascular Drug Therapy*, 2nd edition. W.B. Saunders Co., Philadelphia, 1996, pp 681–689.

51. Carruthers SG. Adverse effects of alpha 1-adrenergic blocking drugs. *Drug Saf* 1994; 11:12–20.

52. Bauer JH, Jones LB, Gaddy P. Effects of prazosin therapy on blood pressure, renal function, and body fluid composition. *Arch Intern Med* 1984; 114:1196–1200.

53. Shabsigh R. Therapy of ED: PDE-5 Inhibitors. *Endocrine* 2004; 23:135–141.

54. Marshall HJ, Beevers DG. Alpha-adrenoceptor blocking drugs and female urinary incontinence: prevalence and reversibility. *Br J Clin Pharmacol* 1996; 42:507–509.

Abbreviations

5-HT	5-hydroxytryptamine / serotonin
AASK	African-American Study of Kidney Disease and Hypertension
ABCD	Appropriate Blood Pressure Control in NIDDM trial
ABPM	ambulatory blood pressure monitoring
ACC	American College of Cardiology
ACCOMPLISH	Avoiding Cardiovascular Events through Combination Therapy in Patients Living with Systolic Hypertension
ACCORD	Action to Control Cardiovascular Risk in Diabetes trial
ACE	angiotensin converting enzyme
ACSM	American College of Sports Medicine
ADHD	attention deficit hyperactivity disorder
AHA	American Heart Association
AIPRI	ACE Inhibition in Progressive Renal Disease Study Group
AKI	acute kidney injury
ALLHAT	Antihypertensive and Lipid-Lowering Treatment to Prevent Heart Attack Trial
ANBP2	Second Australian National Blood Pressure Study
ARB	angiotensin receptor blocker
ARIC	Atherosclerosis Risk in Communities study
AT_1	angiotensin II type I
AT_2	angiotensin II type II
AUA	American Urologic Association
AUR	acute urinary retention
AVOID	Aliskiren in the Evaluation of proteinuria in Diabetes trial
BENEDICT	Bergamo Nephrologic Diabetes Mellitus Complications Trial
BMI	body mass index
BP	blood pressure
BPH	benign prostatic hyperplasia
BUN	blood urea nitrogen
Ca^{2+}	calcium
CAD	coronary artery disease
CARDIA	Coronary Artery Risk Development in Young Adults
CCB	calcium channel blocker
CDC	Center for Disease Control
CHD	coronary heart disease
CHF	congestive heart failure
CHS	Cardiovascular Health Study
CI	confidence interval
CIMT	carotid artery intimal-medial thickness
CKD	chronic kidney disease
CNS	central nervous system

COOPERATE	Combination Treatment of Angiotensin Receptor Blocker and Angiotensin Converting Enzyme Inhibitor in Non-diabetic Renal Disease trial
CT	computed tomographic
CV	cardiovascular
CVD	cardiovascular disease
D2	dopamine 2 receptor
D/C	doxazosin compared to chlorthalidone
DAPHNE	Doxazosin Atherosclerosis Progression Study in Hypertensives
DASH	Dietary Approaches to Stop Hypertension
DBP	diastolic blood pressure
DEW-IT	Diet, Exercise and Weight-loss Intervention Trial
DM	diabetes mellitus
DMSA	dimercaptosuccunic acid
eGFR	estimated glomerular filtration rate
EPHESUS	Eplerenone Post-Acute Myocardial Infarction Heart Failure Efficacy and Survival Study
ESC	European Society of Cardiology
ESCAPE-2	Efficacy Study of Clevidipine Assessing its Postoperative Antihypertensive Effect in Cardiac Surgery-2 trial
ESH	European Society of Hypertension
ESRD	end-stage renal disease
EWPHBPE	European Working Party on High Blood Pressure in the Elderly
FSA	Food Standards Agency(UK)
GABA	gamma-aminobutyric acid
GEMINI	Glycemic Effects in Diabetes Mellitus Carvedilol-Metoprolol Comparison in Hypertensives trial
GFR	glomerular filtration rate
GISEN	Gruppo Italiano di Studi Epidemiologici in Nefrologia
H1	histamine 1 receptor
HCTZ	hydrochlorothiazide
HDFP	Hypertension Detection and Follow-up Program
HDL	high density lipoprotein
HF	heart failure
HOPE	Heart Outcomes Prevention Evaluation trial
HOT	Hypertension Optimal Treatment trial
HR	heart rate
hs-CRP	high sensitivity C-reactive protein
HTN	hypertension
HYVET	Hypertension in the Very Elderly Trial
IDNT	Irbesartan in Diabetic Nephropathy Trial
IHD	ischemic heart disease
IMT	intimal-medial thickness
INSIGHT	International Nifedipine GITS Study
ISH	isolated systolic hypertension
IV	intravenous
JNC	Joint National Committee on Prevention, Detection, Evaluation and Treatment of High Blood Pressure
K^+	potassium
KEEP	Kidney Early Evaluation Program
KDOQI	Kidney Disease Outcome Quality Initiative
LDL	low density lipoprotein
LUTS	lower urinary tract symptom

LV	left ventricular
LVH	left ventricular hypertrophy
LVM	left ventricular mass
MAO	monoamine oxidase
MAP	mean arterial pressure
MAPHY	Metoprolol Atherosclerosis Prevention in Hypertensives
MAXO$_2$	maximal oxygen uptake
MDRD	Modification of Diet in Renal Disease
MERIT-HF	Metoprolol CR/XL Randomized Intervention Trial in congestive Heart Failure
Mg^{2+}	magnesium
MI	myocardial infarction
MIDAS	Multicenter Isradipine Diuretic Atherosclerosis Study
MR	modified release
MRA	magnetic resonance angiography
MRC	Medical Research Council
MRFIT	Multiple Risk Factor Intervention Trial
MRI	magnetic resonance imaging
MTOPS	Medical Therapy of Prostatic Symptoms trial
MVC	maximal voluntary contraction
NaCl	sodium chloride
NE	norepinephrine
NFK	National Kidney Foundation
NHANES	National Health and Nutrition Examination Survey
NHBPEP	National High Blood Pressure Education Program
NSAID	non-steroidal anti-inflammatory drug
OCAS	oral controlled absorption system
OCD	obsessive compulsive disorder
OH	orthostatic hypotension
OTC	over-the-counter
PLESS	Proscar™ (finasteride) Long-Term Efficacy and Safety Study
PNS	parasympathetic nervous system
PP	pulse pressure
PPE	pre-participation physical evaluation
PVR	peripheral vascular resistance
RAAS	renin angiotensin-aldosterone system
RAS	renin-angiotensin system
RBC	red blood cell
RCT	randomized controlled trial
REASON	Preterax in Regression of Arterial Stiffness in a Controlled Double-Blind study
REIN	Ramipril Efficacy In Nephropathy trial
RENAAL	Reduction of Endpoints in NIDDM with the Angiotensin II Antagonist Losartan study
RPE	rating of perceived exertion
RR	risk ratio
SBP	systolic blood pressure
SHEP	Systolic Hypertension in the Elderly
SI	Special Intervention
SNRI	serotonin-norepinephrine reuptake inhibitor
SNS	sympathetic nervous system
SSH	spurious systolic hypertension

SSRI	serotonin reuptake inhibitor
STAR	Study of Trandolapril/Verapamil SR And Insulin Resistance
Syst-Eur	Systolic Hypertension in Europe
TCA	tricyclic antidepressant
TM	Transcendental Meditation
TOMHS	Treatment of Mild Hypertension Study
TOPH	Trials of Hypertension Prevention
TURP	transurethral prostatectomy
UACR	urinary albumin:creatinine
UAE	urine albumin excretion
UC	Usual Care
UKPDS	United Kingdom Prospective Diabetes Study
VA	Veterans Affairs
VLDL	very low density lipoprotein
WCH	white coat hypertension